The Cancer Prevention Good Health Diet

BOOKS BY MARTIN KATAHN, PH.D.

The 200 Calorie Solution

Beyond Diet

The Rotation Diet

The Rotation Diet Cookbook
(with Terri Katahn)

The T-Factor Diet

The T-Factor Fat Gram Counter
(with Jamie Pope)

One Meal at a Time

The Low-Fat Supermarket Guide
(with Jamie Pope)

The Low-Fat Fast Food Guide
(with Jamie Pope)

The Low-Fat Good Food Cookbook
(with Terri Katahn)

How to Quit Smoking without Gaining Weight

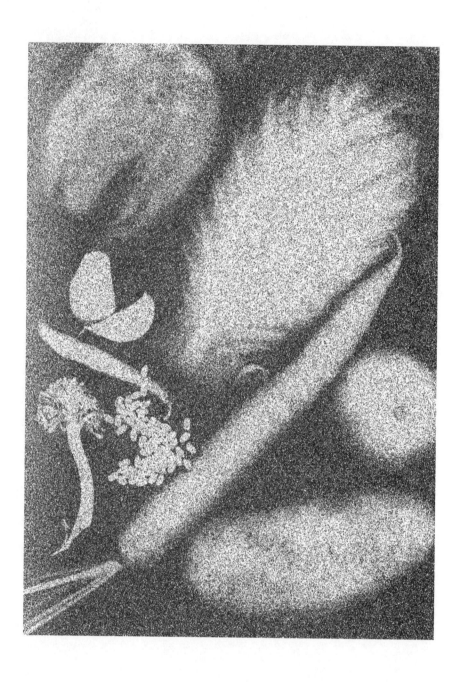

The Cancer Prevention Good Health Diet

A Complete Program for a Longer, Healthier Life

Martin Katahn, Ph.D.

W · W · Norton & Company   New York · London

For information about permission to reproduce selections from this book, write to Permissions,
W. W. Norton & Company, Inc., 500 Fifth Avenue, New York, N.Y. 10110.

The text of this book is composed in 11/13 Berkeley Book with tables in Futura Light and Medium.
The display is set in Slimline Bold with Berkeley Bold and Medium.
Composition and manufacturing by The Haddon Craftsmen, Inc.
Book design by Margaret M. Wagner.

Originally published under the title The Tri-Color Diet.

ISBN 0-393-32058-8

W. W. Norton & Company, Inc., 500 Fifth Avenue, New York, N.Y. 10110
www.wwnorton.com
W. W. Norton & Company Ltd., 10 Coptic Street, London WC1A 1PU

1 2 3 4 5 6 7 8 9 0

Contents

Acknowledgments

I could never have finished this book anywhere near its target date nor could I have illustrated how to make a healthful plant-food-based diet tasty and attractive to many people who "don't like veggies" without the help of my wife, Enid. In spite of having to maintain her own full-time career as a pianist, she took charge of creating and preparing the majority of recipes in this book, and testing all of them. Thank you very much.

Special thanks go to Dr. Lee Fleshood, formerly director of nutrition in the Department of Health and Human Services of the state of Tennessee, for showing up at my doorstep at 7:00 A.M. on Saturday mornings with packets of articles to help keep me up to date on the latest research and for the discussions that followed during the hour that we walked around the neighborhood.

Thanks also to the many friends and colleagues who gave me their own favorite plant-food recipes or who, without prior knowledge of what to expect, tasted and gave me their opinions about the recipes that ended up in this book: Tony Belcher, Burnetta Clayton, Dr. Ford Ebner, Inka Goel, Dr. Fred Goldner, Martha Goldner, Dr. Carl Haywood, Dona Haywood, Monna Journey, David Katahn, Starling Lawrence, Reyna Thera Lorele, Maureen Needham, Richard Odom, Richard Pine, Dr. Maureen Powers, Dr. Phil Schoggen, Dikkie Schoggen, Dr. Bill Smith, Dr. Leslie Smith, Dr. Ruth Smith, Dr. Hans Strupp, Lottie Strupp, and Lee Wilson.

Once again, many thanks to these folks, some of whom have been working with me for the past fifteen years: my agent, Richard Pine, and director of subsidiary rights, Lori Andiman, and the team at W. W. Norton that helped me put this book together: my editor, Starling Lawrence; manuscript editor, Debra Makay; production manager, Andrew Marasia; editorial assistant, Patricia Chui; and managing editor, Nancy Palmquist.

Preface

Over 1200 reports on the relationship between nutritional factors and cancer have appeared in the research literature since the publication of the first edition of this book. The evidence is now even more overwhelming: *by switching to a plant-based diet, cutting back on your fat consumption (especially saturated fat) and limiting your consumption of red meat, you can cut your risk of cancer (and heart disease) by 50 to 80 percent.*

I'm quite sure you have heard this kind of advice before. But if you have failed to put it into practice, it may be because you found that it was inconvenient to plan and prepare a plant-based diet. In addition to the inconvenience, you may not have been able to design a more healthful diet that could also give you the gustatory satisfaction that you obtained from your customary way of eating.

My primary objective in this book is to make good health taste good. Cancer prevention does not require that you become an ascetic. Every recipe in this book was created by my wife or myself, or tested by us and our friends, to make sure it would have wide appeal. If you give these recipes and menus an honest try, within a few short weeks I think you will notice some significant changes. I think you will find that preparing more healthful foods gets easier and easier and that your tastes will change. Best of all, you can be confident that by making these changes, you have at least doubled the likelihood of adding many healthy years to your life.

To help interested readers who are not cancer specialists become more familiar with the latest research, I have added a number of key journal articles to Appendix A from among the hundreds that have appeared since the first edition of this book. These studies, with their reference lists, can guide you to a comprehensive review of the entire literature.

Introduction

How would you like to add as much as 20 years or more of disease-free living to your life? No cancer. No heart disease. Just pure, unadulterated, good health.

The means of doubling, even tripling, your chances of doing this lie squarely in your own hands. It begins with diet.

The Background

For the past several years evidence has been accumulating that the human body depends upon more than just the well-known vitamins and minerals to stay healthy. Scientists have discovered that it may take hundreds, possibly even thousands, of different food compounds called *phytochemicals* to maintain our immune systems at maximum strength and protect us from cancer and atherosclerosis, as well as other degenerative diseases.

These substances are called phytochemicals because they are found *only* in plants (*phyto* comes from the Greek word for "plant"). The discovery of the various ingredients in plants that appear to be *absolutely essential* in maximizing our resistance to cancer and heart disease has been hailed as a nutritional breakthrough equal in importance to the discovery earlier in this century of the role that vitamins and minerals play in promoting growth and maintaining good health. Inadequate representation of these compounds in the typical American diet may be the main nutritional factor underlying the high rate of premature, unnecessary, and avoidable heart disease and cancer in this country. And the reason the same plant compounds and the same healthful diet protect against both cancer and heart disease is that these two illnesses share similar causes and characteristics. That is, the same dangerous biochemical and physiological events that can result in cancer when they occur in various body organs and tissues may lead to atherosclerosis when they occur in your bloodstream and arterial walls.

The Cancer Prevention Good Health Diet: Primary Objectives

My first objective in *The Cancer Prevention Good Health Diet* has three parts. I want to explain (1) what these phytochemicals are, (2) why and how they can protect you against both cancer and heart disease, and (3) where to find them in different fruits, vegetables, nuts, seeds, and commonly used spices and herbs.

There are literally thousands of different phytochemicals (one of my reference books lists over 20,000, although the total number present in plants is probably considerably greater than that). In addition to certain vitamins and trace minerals, the specific phytochemicals that appear to play key roles in the prevention of cancer and heart disease fall into several main groups based on their chemical structure: phenols, thiols, carotenoids and retinoids, terpenes, tocopherols, isothiocyanates, indoles, dithiothiones, and polyacetylenes, among others. Research at the present time suggests that representation from many if not all of the different groups may be important to our health. Fortunately, important groups of phytochemicals often occur together in individual plant foods, or in combinations of foods that make for excellent recipes. I'll give you the key to this grouping in *The Cancer Prevention Good Health Diet.*

My second objective may be even more important than the first. Although the Cancer Prevention Good Health Diet may add many healthy years to your life, I know that if you don't like my recommendations and find them easy to follow, no matter how much good they might do, you won't stick with them and the whole effort will have been wasted. So I promise you that the Cancer Prevention Good Health Diet will make good health taste good. In fact, I think that following this diet is going to give you such culinary enjoyment and gustatory pleasure that you will never consider going back to a diet that has, perhaps without your awareness, been killing you.

Have you been eating yourself into an early grave?

It really is true. If you have been eating the typical American diet, there is a good chance you have been eating yourself into an early, painful, and costly battle with cancer, heart disease, or some other degenerative disease such as high blood pressure, adult-onset diabetes, or arthritis. The diet eaten by the average American is prematurely killing more people each year than have died in all wars that we have fought since the founding of our country!

Not only is our typical diet seriously lacking in many of the plant-based nutrients and phytochemicals that can help sustain our health throughout our lives, but it is chock-full of exactly the things that encourage the development of the killer diseases: *too much fat, too many calories* (especially the empty, sugar-laden kind), and *too much red meat.* Together with our sedentary lifestyle, this diet is also a major factor in the epidemic of obesity in this country. Fully one-third of the population is so overweight as to make their weight an independent contributing factor to just about every known degenerative disease from cancer and heart disease to hypertension, diabetes, and arthritis.

I'll explain in greater detail at relevant points in this book how the typical American diet can be robbing you of many years of good health by fostering the early onset of cancer and heart disease. But more important than these explanations is the remedy—the Cancer Prevention Good Health Diet.

What Is the Cancer Prevention Good Health Diet?

Because some of the most important protective phytochemicals actually give foods their distinctive colors, color plays a key role in the Cancer Prevention Good Health Diet. Each time you eat a slice of tomato, a spoonful of cantaloupe, or a forkful of a leafy green vegetable, you are consuming a different group of phytochemicals, each of which can have a different "chemopreventive" role to play. Some neutralize carcinogenic substances before they can attack your body cells. Others kill cancer cells before they can multiply or prevent damage to your circulatory system that can lead to atherosclerosis. In fact, each of these different plant foods contains a whole array of different phytochemicals, possibly numbering in the thousands, and experts now believe that it may take hundreds of them, *working together* and in conjunction with different vitamins and minerals, to guard you against diseases of all kinds in addition to cancer and heart disease. I emphasize "working together" because they appear to depend on each other in the amounts and in the relationships that are found in the plant foods themselves. You can obtain this kind of protection only from your diet—NOT FROM ANY KIND OF SUPPLEMENT OR PILL. I will discuss the pros and cons of supplementation in Chapter 8.

The color of your fruits and vegetables—red, yellow/orange, green—is an important part of the Cancer Prevention Good Health Diet because it provides you with a key to certain essential food choices. But this is only part of the wonderful and fascinating story of how plants developed mechanisms for protecting themselves from disease and other dangers in their environments, and how, when we human beings appeared on the scene, many of the chemicals involved in plant health became essential to our own. I'll tell you more about this in Chapter 3.

It's obvious by now that I'm going to be encouraging you to eat more fruits and vegetables, as well as other plant foods. I suspect that you may have heard this advice so often it may have a tendency to go in one ear and out the other. So you're probably wondering what's different about the Cancer Prevention Good Health Diet. As you will discover, certain foods contain concentrations of different phytochemicals with different disease-fighting powers. *The Cancer Prevention Good Health Diet* will provide you with the information you need to cover all the bases as only diet, not pills, can do.

A Promise

After showing you what you need to know, my main emphasis will be on how to put your knowledge into practice. And to this purpose I promise: *no feelings of deprivation!* My ultimate goal is to demonstrate, with over a hundred different, unbelievably delicious recipes, that you can make eating "right" taste just as good as eating "wrong," and that you can make these potentially life-saving changes in a way that's incredibly easy and convenient. No drastic, overnight changes are required. You go at your own pace, discovering new ways to prepare and combine healthful foods *one recipe, one meal, one day at a time.*

If you have a few pounds to lose, they're almost certain to fall away gradually, *without your making any special effort.* And those pounds lost will stay lost! There are no difficult formulas to follow and no calculations or record keeping (not of calories, not even fat grams, unless there is a special reason for you to lose a lot of weight in a hurry or unless that sort of record keeping appeals to you). The Cancer Prevention Good Health Diet is a very natural diet with just a few simple guidelines. And everything you need can be found at your favorite supermarket.

But now, let's talk a little more about your weight, because THINNER REALLY IS BETTER!

In 1990 the U.S. Department of Agriculture (USDA) and the U.S. Department of Health and Human Services (DHHS) revised their previous recommendations and added as much as 10 to 20 pounds across the board in the table of suggested weights included in the bulletin *Nutrition and Your Health: Dietary Guidelines for Americans*. This increase was immediately and widely criticized by many health experts, who pointed out that the research on which it was based was flawed. How right they were.[1]

In fact, the 1990 guidelines are so inflated they may be downright dangerous.

Many studies have shown that at least one-third of the incidence of heart disease and cancer is weight related. But, until recently, many experts felt that the risk did not increase significantly until people were considerably above *average* weight. Just-published results of two very large ongoing studies, the Nurses' Health Study and the Physicians' Health Study,[2] now show that *even a little bit of excess weight* can put you at a seriously increased risk not only for heart disease and certain cancers, but for something so far removed from weight in most people's minds as cataracts. These studies show that persons of *average weight* in the United States are *about 15 to 20 percent above the weight* that would put them at the lowest risk for all of these illnesses.

For example, if you are a woman of average height (5-foot-5), the weight associated with the least risk of heart disease is a mere 119 pounds. Fewer than 13 percent of American women over the age of 35 can boast of meeting this weight criterion, which is actually 7 pounds *below* the *lowest* weight (126 pounds) in the 1990 federal table of suggested weights. Women of average weight, which ranges between 150 and 160 pounds and falls within federal guidelines, have a 30 percent greater risk. If you are a 5-foot-10 man, the weight associated with the least risk of cataracts is a lean 153 pounds. The risk increases with added weight until, at 193 pounds, it's doubled. Only about 12 percent of men meet the lean criterion, which is about 25 pounds below the midpoint of the range that is suggested in the federal guidelines for a man of that height over 35 years old.

If you are an overweight person and have any interest in preserving your health, this recent research may motivate you to shed a little weight. But before you go off on an almost-certain-to-fail fad diet in an effort to lose your extra pounds, you should consider these facts:

[1] Smokers, who weigh less on average than non-smokers but who die younger, were included in establishing the suggested weights, thus making it appear that being heavier was healthier. In addition, it is also possible that persons already ill without knowing it, and lighter as a result, were included in the calculations.

[2] I will normally avoid giving details of particular studies in the main text of this book. Please refer to Appendix A for a list of references and a discussion of the research on which *The Cancer Prevention Good Health Diet* is based.

Between 90 and 95 percent of people who go on quick-weight-loss diets gain all their weight back within a year or two, and often with a few extra pounds. And repeatedly going on diets—losing and regaining weight—may hasten the progression of the atherosclerotic process and be even more dangerous to your health than staying fat!

The main reasons most people fail to achieve permanent weight loss are split about evenly between genetic and behavioral factors.

Genetic Contributions to Obesity

The more overweight you are, the more likely genetic influences are playing an important role and making it much harder for you to reach your healthiest weight than it is for the average person. The activity of certain genes may make it harder for you to control your appetite while other genes may make it easier for your body to put fat into storage. Still other genes determine where the major part of that fat will go on your body, and if they prefer hips, buttocks, and thighs, rather than the upper parts of the body for storage, it may be especially hard to rid yourself of the excess. And still other genes may be putting a damper on your metabolic rate so that, throughout the day, both at rest and during physical activity, you burn fewer calories than the average person.

If you have been fighting a losing battle with your weight, these genetic factors raise the question: "Are you destined to be fat?"

The Setpoint

Some experts have suggested that these and still other genetic factors establish a setpoint for your weight and that efforts to lose weight are almost always destined to fail. They claim that your body works very hard to adjust both its metabolic rate and its rate of fat storage until it returns to a preferred, predetermined percentage of body fat. *This is simply not true.*

The setpoint for body weight is not a point! It's a *range*.

Your behavior can combat and, to a certain extent, actually alter inherited metabolic tendencies. All of us, no matter how strong our genetic predispositions, have a range in which our weight can vary depending on our lifestyle. All it takes to be at the top or bottom of that range are moderate changes in diet and physical activity. In other words, you can permanently reset your setpoint to be at the top or bottom of your range. Downward changes of as much as 50 to 60 pounds do not require heroic efforts, only some intelligent planning and commitment. But, face it, they do require change! If you sit around all day and eat a high-fat diet, you will be at the top of your range. Get active and follow the Cancer Prevention Good Health Diet, and you will be at the bottom of your range—and for good!

The Cancer Prevention Good Health Diet Also Promises Permanent Weight Management

The Cancer Prevention Good Health Diet is not an "on-again/off-again" diet. It's a diet for life. It leads to a gradual *and permanent* weight loss in virtually all overweight persons. But if you've got more than a few pounds to lose, I'm sure you've got a question:

HOW FAST WILL I LOSE WEIGHT?

You have a choice. You lose weight either way—one slow, one fast. *Both ultimately lead to the same, healthier result.* Which way you choose depends on your health needs and personal preferences.

The Slow Way: A gradual weight loss occurs just by following the guidelines for the prevention of heart disease and cancer that I lay out for you in Chapters 4 and 5. But because it's a one-recipe, one-meal, one-day-at-a-time plan, it's impossible to predict the rate of weight loss. The more you get into the program, the faster it goes, without your having to make any special effort. It requires no calculations—you don't count fat grams or calories—and no record keeping. It's a very easy, leisurely, and convenient way to go about it. If you are a sedentary person and add to the Cancer Prevention Good Health Diet a healthful amount of physical activity, you will gradually reach the weight that is best for you. You will be at the bottom of your setpoint range.

The Fast Way: If you have considerable weight to lose—for example, if you are more than 20 percent over the weight for your height in Table 6.1 (page 73)—the increased risk for heart disease and certain cancers is rather great. And from a psychological perspective, I imagine you'd feel better about yourself if you lost a few pounds. So I am very sympathetic if you want to see some visible progress as quickly as possible. But if you have used a quick-weight-loss plan before, gone off it, and regained some or all of the pounds you lost, I hope you are convinced that that way won't work.

The method you use to lose weight must incorporate exactly the sound nutritional principles you plan to follow for the rest of your life. There must be harmony between the way you go about losing weight and the way you will ultimately maintain your lower weight. New taste preferences and methods of food preparation, and, if you are a sedentary person, increased physical activity, must become fully ingrained in your life *as you lose your weight*. Nothing changes when you reach your goal weight except that you can be more relaxed about eating the foods you have already learned to enjoy.

In order to help you lose weight as quickly as possible in a healthful way, and at the same time help ensure that you will achieve permanent weight management, I have designed the Weight-Loss Express.

Some Bonuses

Whether or not you are overweight I know that if you follow the Cancer Prevention Good Health Diet you will feel better than you have felt in a long time. You will be more comfortable after eating, you will have more energy, and you will sleep better. As an end result, I think you will like yourself better because you will know that by doing everything you can for your own health, you are doing something good for the people in your life who love you and depend on you.

To give you some additional, if not traditional, advice on how to complete your program of disease prevention, I also will review recent evidence showing that a number of the plants used for hundreds of years as folk medicines in our own culture, as well as in Far Eastern and so-called primitive cultures, have clear anticarcinogenic and other medicinal activity when included in the diet. However, other plants are useless, and some are dangerous. I will present this information together with my recommendations in Chapter 8. Many of the useful and safe plant products are already available in your supermarket or, if not there, in a local health-food store.

Finally, although diet is the cornerstone, there is more to a healthful, disease-prevention lifestyle than diet alone. In Chapter 9 I'll discuss the importance of physical activity in the prevention of disease and for permanent weight management. If you are a sedentary person, I'll show you "how to succeed in becoming an active person without really trying." I'll also show you how to reduce stress and give you advice on how to deal with cancer-causing agents in your environment.

And now, I hope that *The Cancer Prevention Good Health Diet* will put you on the path to a thinner, happier, healthier, and longer life.

The Cancer Prevention Good Health Diet

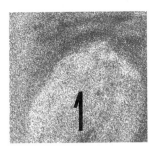

What Is Cancer and What Causes It?

Odds are about 1 in 3 that the average American will end up developing some form of cancer. Some 1.2 million Americans did in 1995, and over 500,000 died. Both figures have been increasing, year after year.

The odds that the average American will ultimately develop some form of cardiovascular disease are about double those for cancer, and each year almost twice as many people die from cardiovascular disease as from cancer.

Perhaps the most tragic thing about this situation is that so much of this illness and early mortality (before the age of 65) is needless. It can be avoided. Experts estimate that between 50 and 80 percent of the premature incidence of illness and death from cancer and cardiovascular disease is due, to put it bluntly, to a lousy lifestyle. It could be cut in half. Of course, there's no absolute guarantee that you or any other particular individual will never develop cancer or heart disease, but the odds that it might happen to you can be reduced at least by half, and perhaps by more, if you will just follow the advice I'm about to give you.

Your first line of defense against cancer and heart disease is your diet.

Some of the things you eat actually promote the development of cancer and heart disease, while others prevent it. Every time you bring your fork to your mouth, you have a hand in deciding whether you will enjoy your maximum "health span"—that is, the full allotment of *healthy* years of life that's stored in your genetic potential—or you will self-destruct before your time. It can mean a difference of 5, 10, 20, or even more years of good health, instead of suffering and doctor bills.

Because cancer is such a dreaded disease many people tend to shy away from thinking about the possibility that they might become a victim themselves, often until it's too late to take the steps that might have prevented it. But I think that the more you understand the nature of the disease and the very potent steps you can take to prevent it, the more motivated you will be to eliminate all possible lifestyle risks.

So, in this chapter I want to explain what cancer is and what causes it. I'll discuss the influence of heredity, and the roles played by diet and other lifestyle factors. In Chapter 2, I'll describe some of the ways in which cancer and atherosclerosis are similar diseases, caused by similar physiological events. Then, in Chapter 3, I will explain how phytochemicals and antioxidant components in your food do double duty, blocking or suppressing both cancerous growths and the progression of heart disease.

Time is on your side!

Since most cancers lie sleeping in your body for 10 to 30 years before they wake up and become active, it's not too late to suppress their development while they are still asleep. And, compared with cancer, it may take even longer for heart disease to reach life-threatening proportions. I hope my explanations in the following pages will convince you that you can do a great deal to stop cancer and heart disease dead in their tracks and that the Cancer Prevention Good Health Diet can be your nutritional ally.

What Is Cancer and What Causes It?

Cancer is not a single disease. There are about 200 different kinds of cancer and they can occur anywhere in your body. However, all forms of cancer share a distinguishing characteristic. They all begin when internal command centers in a body cell become damaged and the cell loses both the ability to reproduce itself in a controlled way and the ability to carry out the original, proper functions of the tissue in which it originated. The damaged cell passes along this inability to control its reproductive function to each daughter cell, and the uncontrolled, disorganized growth of these cells begins to proceed geometrically: 1 cell becomes 2, 2 become 4, 4 become 8, and so on. This explosive growth can result in what is called a *malignant* (injurious or destructive) tumor, that is, a cancer.

Not all tumors are cancerous, however. Most are benign—they remain localized, grow slowly, and tend to resemble the tissue of origin. They tend to be encapsulated and do not invade surrounding tissues or organs, although they may endanger a person by exerting harmful pressure on neighboring parts of the body, such as in the brain. Some benign tumors may, however, become cancerous, such as polyps of the colon.

A malignant tumor, in contrast, can interfere with the proper functioning of the part of the body where it originated, or it may pierce the boundaries of the tissue where it first started, spread out, and interfere with the function of a neighboring organ. After a time, cancer cells may *metastasize;* that is, some of them may break away from their original site and travel to distant parts of the body via the bloodstream or lymph system. This can result in new malignant growths in other tissues and body organs. In the end, one or more of these growths can cause a vital organ to fail and death is the result.

The many different kinds of cancer are grouped into three major categories, depending on the tissue and type of cell from which they originated:

Sarcomas can develop in connective and supportive tissue, such as blood vessels, bone, cartilage, fat, muscle, or nerves.

Carcinomas, the most frequent form of cancer, can develop in epithelial, or covering, tissue, such as the skin, or in the membranes that line body cavities and organs. They also may develop in glandular tissue, such as the breast or prostate. "Adenocarcinoma" is the name given to glandular kinds of cancer, while "squamous-cell carcinoma" refers to skinlike, or scaly, kinds of cancer.

Leukemias and **lymphomas** include cancers that develop in blood-forming tissue, and may result in enlargement of lymph nodes, invasion of the spleen and bone marrow, and the uncontrolled production of immature white blood cells. (Some specialists classify lymphomas in a separate, or fourth, group of cancers.)

The most significant characteristic of a malignant tumor, compared with a benign tumor, is its ability to spread beyond the point of origin. After piercing the surface of the organ in which it originates and entering a body cavity, cells may break away from the parent tumor and become implanted on a neighboring organ. Or they may migrate to the lymph system and end up in the lymph nodes. Some may enter the bloodstream and get carried along until they reach blood vessels that are too small for them to pass through. They get stuck there and continue their multiplication at that point. Tumors originating in the gastrointestinal system tend to migrate first to the liver and later to the lungs, while tumors originating outside the gastrointestinal system tend to go to the lungs first before going on to other organs. This accounts for why so many *metastases*, or secondary growths, occur in the liver and lungs.

GENETIC AND ENVIRONMENTAL INFLUENCES

Between 85 and 90 percent of all cancers can be traced to lifestyle and other environmental causes. Only a few rare kinds of cancer, comprising a very small percentage of all cancers, can be directly attributed to a particular, inherited, defective gene. However, experts believe that complex hereditary factors can influence our *degree of susceptibility* to cancer. This is demonstrated in the way that certain cancers appear to run in families. Here are some examples, with the relative risk factors compared with families in which the disease is not present in siblings or parents:

- Having a parent or sibling with colorectal cancer triples the chance that an individual will also develop the disease.
- A woman having a mother or sister with breast or ovarian cancer has about double the risk for each of these diseases.
- A man having a father or brother with prostate cancer has more than double the risk.

There are about 200 familial patterns that suggest a greater or lesser predisposition to develop different cancers. Although certain shared behavioral factors, such as smoking or working in a similar hazardous job, may play a role in familial patterns, the fact that so many familial patterns for different cancers have been discovered makes the evidence for hereditary influences very convincing.

If you have a parent or sibling who has cancer, or more than one close relative, I want to stress, first, *the importance of discussing this fact with your doctor.* He or she can recommend simple screening procedures that can detect cancer before any symptoms appear to alert you that something is wrong. Except for notable exceptions such as cancers of the lung, liver, and pancreas, *there is an 85 to 99 percent cure rate for most other cancers if they are detected early, while still localized.*

Second, if someone in your immediate family (parent or sibling), or a close relative (aunt, uncle, or grandparent), has developed cancer, this may mean that you carry a heightened susceptibility for that or some other form of cancer. It is obviously important for you to take every possible step you can to prevent cancer from developing before it gains an irreversible foothold. That's where the Cancer Prevention Good Health Diet and other aspects of your lifestyle come in.

Lifestyle factors—that is, our personal behaviors—account for the vast majority of cancers that can be attributed to environmental influences. *The combination of an unhealthy diet and cigarette smoking causes two-thirds of these cancers.* Having an early start in sexual behavior, having many sexual partners, and overindulgence in alcohol account for another 10 percent. Environmental pollution, including radon, automobile exhaust, and industrial hazards, is a leading cause of the rest.

HOW CANCER GETS ITS START IN THE HUMAN BODY

Each of our approximately 75 *trillion* body cells contains 50,000 or more genes in its nucleus. The various configurations and activities of these genes in the different cells of our bodies determine all of our physical and biochemical characteristics, some in an absolute sense, such as the color of our eyes, and some in a way that interacts with our behavior and other environmental factors, such as the ultimate, underlying power of our immune systems to ward off disease.

Certain of the genes in each cell also determine the rate at which that cell will divide and become two. Other genes cooperate to make sure that each new daughter cell is an exact replica of the parent, and that each new cell can do exactly the same job that the parent did in the tissue where it originated. Lung cells are programmed to reproduce lung cells, liver cells make new liver cells, and so on. The daughter cells carry the same program for reproduction in their genes as the parent.

The genes are made up of DNA (deoxyribonucleic acid). The blueprint for all the work that the genes must do is embedded in the DNA. Present research has detected about 60 genes that are active in controlling cellular reproduction (more are continually being discovered). Some are responsible for promoting the division and growth of new cells, while others act as supervisors and repairmen, stopping division and growth at the appropriate time and making repairs in case any mistakes in copying the genetic blueprint have been made. And mistakes can happen.

Considering that an astronomical number of cell replications take place each day (it's in the millions), it's easy to imagine that, just by chance, a copying error can occur. By analogy, it's a bit like you or me making a certain number of mistakes if we tried to copy a dictionary, word for word, with all the punctuation marks exactly right. Normally, however, the genes responsible for catching mistakes and repairing them stop the replication process and the growth of the new daughter cell while other genes send out enzymes to correct the error. Repairs are sometimes not successful, however, and the daughter cell does end up carrying an incorrect blueprint. When this occurs, yet other genes can detect that failure and cause the changed or *mutated* cell that carries a defective gene or genes to self-destruct before it begins to divide and replicate. These activities are just part of an even more elaborate defense system that goes to work to protect the DNA from damage by carcinogenic substances, as well as to ensure the replication of cells without the kind of damage that might lead to cancer.

Initiation and Promotion in the Development of Cancer

There are, as you are probably well aware, many cancer-causing, or carcinogenic, substances in our environment. They're called *carcinogenic* because they have the ability to penetrate cell walls and damage the DNA that contains the blueprint for cellular reproduction. These substances include cigarette smoke, air pollution (such as automobile exhaust), pesticides in our food, various drugs and industrial chemicals, ultraviolet radiation, X-rays, and certain viruses, among others. Now, among those many genes that normally play a useful role in cell growth and division are some called *proto-oncogenes* (*onco* comes from a Greek word meaning "mass" or "tumor," and *proto* from one meaning "before" or "giving rise to"). Should one of these be damaged, it can become hyperactive and changed into an *oncogene* that may then begin the transformation of that cell into a cancer cell.

This one event, while it may *initiate* the cancerous process, will, by itself, rarely if ever cause cancer. A cell with a defective gene can lie dormant throughout a person's lifetime. To develop into an active, growing, and replicating cancer cell usually requires many years of "encouragement" from other substances called *promoters*. Promoters by themselves (just like initiators all by themselves) don't cause cancer. Promoters become dangerous only after a cell has already been damaged by an initiator that created one or more defective genes. Promoters stimulate defective (initiated) genes to express themselves, and, ultimately, after the body's defenses are exhausted, defective genes begin to express themselves without restraint, causing uncontrolled the cell division.

Cigarette smoke provides a good example of the process, all by itself. It contains many chemical promoters as well as initiators. Even though smoking may have initiated the carcinogenic process in one or more of a smoker's lung cells, when a person quits smoking and the defective genes are no longer being egged on to express themselves by the promoters in cigarette smoke, the risk of lung cancer drops quite rapidly.

And it's important to point out that alcohol, which in non-smokers has only slight carcinogenic activity, becomes a very potent promoter of lung cancer when combined with cigarettes. Alcohol combined with smoking doubles the risk of lung cancer from smoking alone.

From a nutritional standpoint, *too much fat* appears to be the most dangerous promoter of almost all kinds of cancer, including colon, prostate, ovarian, uterine, skin, and breast. Saturated fat, found in large quantities in animal products, appears to have a particularly strong role in the development of lung cancer, as well as cancer of the colon, prostate, and breast. I will explain how too much fat in the diet encourages so many different kinds of cancer in Chapter 3.

Carcinogens Have a Common Mechanism of Action

Although many different chemicals can cause cancer, most of them are not capable of it in the form that exists when they first enter a person's body. But they all appear to do it via a common mechanism of action that works in the following way.

As the body tries to rid itself of dangerous substances, it attempts to convert them into a harmless form that can be easily excreted. Unfortunately, along the way, certain by-products of the transformation are created, which appear to have in common some similar molecular structures that enable them to interact with and damage the molecules in cellular membranes and DNA. As a class, these dangerous molecules are sometimes referred to as *electrophilic* because they "love" to steal electrons from other molecules, or bond with them, or break them up in order to latch on to another electron and incorporate it in their own structure.

Free radicals are one kind of electrophilic by-product, and understanding how they can become dangerous will give you an idea of how electrophilic molecules in general play their parts in the potentially carcinogenic process.

Free Radicals and How They Can Harm Your Body

Free radicals are actually created in our bodies in vast numbers every day. Some of them carry out important, lifesaving tasks. For example, when deadly bacteria invade our bodies, our immune systems analyze the chemical pattern of the intruders and create an army of specially designed cells that are actually free radicals. These free radicals have exactly the right chemical structure to bond with and destroy the bacteria before they can kill us. When their work is done, the body ceases production of these disease-fighting free radicals and the system returns to normal.

Free radicals are also created during normal cellular metabolic processes—for example, during the transfer of nutrients and energy, during cell division and replication, and during the disposal of wastes. Both emotional stress and exercise are also known to increase the production of free radicals (which the body can easily handle at moderate levels). And, as you might imagine, they are created when the body tries to eliminate or detoxify carcinogenic environmental substances or their effects: cigarette smoke, alcohol, automobile exhaust and other pollutants in the air, ultraviolet radiation, and petrochemicals and herbicides in food, among others.

So where is the potential for great harm from the common product of all these events?

Free radicals contain an atom with a missing electron. Frequently, the missing electron is in an atom of oxygen. Now, when an atom is missing an electron it is highly unstable or reactive—it wants to connect up with another electron because electrons like to travel in pairs. Therefore, it will attack a nearby molecule and grab one of its electrons. In so doing, it changes the electrochemical characteristics of the target molecule, and it, in turn, having lost an electron, becomes a free radical. And now the newly created free radical goes searching to steal an electron from another molecule.

This process of stealing electrons is called *oxidation.* Free radicals are *oxidants,* and the target molecules are *oxidized.* Normally, when oxidation is sensed, the body immediately creates *antioxidants* to bind with the free radicals, neutralize them, and dispose of them before they can damage critical cellular components.

However, under continual or intense exposure to carcinogenic substances, or if the body's antioxidant supply is less than optimum, the process of free-radical creation may get out of hand and a regular avalanche of free radicals can occur that outruns the body's ability to produce enough antioxidants. Various components within a cell where this is happening may be damaged to the point where they cannot carry out their intended functions. If it occurs in the membrane of a cell, where fatty acids (especially susceptible targets) form about 50 percent of the structure, the membrane may lose its ability to prevent dangerous carcinogenic substances from penetrating into the cell. If a free-radical storm happens within a cell, the DNA may be damaged and the genes responsible for replication may become unable to control the process.

The burden that free radicals put upon the body's defenses contributes to what is called *oxidative stress*. As I mentioned earlier, a number of other electrophilic molecules are created in the body's attempts to dispose of carcinogenic compounds. These molecules have characteristics similar to, and sometimes even more dangerous than, those of the free radicals, but they all share a common characteristic: they are all oxidants that can steal electrons or break up and damage essential cellular components in their attempt to find electron mates. The process is very similar to the way oxygen molecules combine with metal and cause rust or, with the help of heat, bond with molecules of fat or oil and cause them to become rancid. Obviously, the less oxidative stress we create from our lifestyles or from other environmental causes, and the stronger our army of antioxidants to protect us from this kind of damage, the better off we are.

Dietary Antioxidants and Phytochemicals

Although the body creates its own arsenal of antioxidants, certain antioxidants in food, such as vitamins A, C, and E and beta-carotene (which is changed into vitamin A after ingestion), together with certain antioxidant phytochemicals may play essential roles in preventing the oxidation process and the development of cancer. But none of these antioxidants is capable of defending the body against cancer all by itself. And, as I will explain in Chapter 3, there is more to the system of defenses against cancer than just the presence of antioxidants. The most important point of all is that the system of defenses is effective *only when the various essential nutrients and the hundreds and possibly thousands of other supporting phytochemicals are consumed together, as found in real food.* I cannot emphasize enough the importance of your entire diet.

Recent research suggests that atherosclerosis and cancer may share some similar causes and characteristics and that some of the same protective vitamins and phytochemicals that are involved in building your body's defenses against cancer may also protect you from atherosclerosis. This is the topic of the next chapter.

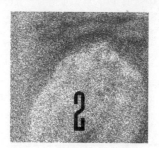

Diet and Cardiovascular Disease

The Problem of Heart Disease: Some Background

Cardiovascular disease claims over a million deaths each year, making it the number-one cause of death among adults in the United States. Medical experts have preached about the importance of a person's lifestyle in the cause of cardiovascular disease for so long that I feel quite certain most health-conscious persons are already well acquainted with the major behavioral risk factors. Although heredity and age, which are out of our control, each contribute to the risk of cardiovascular disease, behavioral factors such as cigarette smoking, too much fat in the diet and a paucity of protective plant foods, lack of physical activity, and obesity can all play key roles in the premature appearance of this disease.

While improvements in medical care have helped reduce mortality from heart disease during the last decade, at least part of the improvement appears to have resulted from lifestyle changes, especially the reduction in cigarette smoking. If you are a cigarette smoker, the very best thing you can do for your health is to join the trend and quit.[1]

With respect to diet, however, the picture is not particularly good. Experts all agree that in order to make a major reduction in the incidence of both cancer and heart disease we must make some major changes in our

[1] If you are a smoker and concerned about weight gain if you quit, I have written a book that can help you: *How to Quit Smoking without Gaining Weight* (W. W. Norton, 1994).

diet. Most recommend reducing fat intake to around 20 percent of total calories.[2] Americans are nowhere close to that. While total fat consumption as a percentage of total calories has reportedly come down a couple of percentage points from 36 to 34 percent, Americans are actually eating 100 to 300 calories more each day.[3] This means that the real amount of fat being consumed, in absolute terms, may be as high as it ever was. And since 60 percent of the U.S. population fails to get even 20 minutes of exercise three times a week, it's no surprise that 1 out of 3 of us is more than 20 percent overweight, which is an all-time high.

As for what may be the most dangerous kind of fat in our diets—*saturated fat*—consumption of saturated fat from certain animal products, such as whole milk, butter, and red meat, has decreased. But consumption of other high-fat animal products has *increased* dramatically—for example, cheese, as well as premium, high-fat ice cream (which is at a peak). So, while the proportion of deaths from cardiovascular disease may have decreased in the total number of deaths that occur each year, our failure to make a real improvement in diet, weight management, and exercise continues to make it the number-one cause of death in the United States.

Serum Cholesterol, Saturated Fat, and Oxidized LDL as Factors in Heart Disease

Elevated serum cholesterol (blood cholesterol levels), especially the low-density-lipoprotein (LDL) component, is an important risk factor for cardiovascular disease. The reason for concern with LDL is that these large, lipid-laden LDL molecules are the ones that accumulate to form atherosclerotic plaque. Both hereditary and behavioral factors influence our cholesterol level.

The National Cholesterol Education Program (NCEP) considers a total serum cholesterol of 200–239 milliliters per decaliter (ml/dl), or an LDL

---

[2]Some experts go so far as to suggest a diet with only 10 percent fat, but virtually no one can stick with such a restrictive diet for any length of time unless the environment permits no free choice, or they are highly motivated research participants.

[3]These figures are based on the recent National Health and Nutrition Survey III. However, when laboratory studies comparing actual caloric needs to maintain a given body weight are compared with the number of calories contained in the amount of food people say they eat in response to survey questions, the studies find that people underestimate their caloric consumption by an average of about 20 percent. The underestimation is due primarily to an inaccurate reporting of fat intake. Thus, the National Health and Nutrition Survey III probably underestimates the true consumption of fat by a considerable amount. It is quite likely that the average American diet contains closer to 40 percent of calories from fat, rather than 34 percent.

component of 130–159 ml/dl, to be borderline high and a reason to take remedial steps with diet and exercise. A total serum cholesterol level of 240 ml/dl and above, or an LDL component of 160 ml/dl and above, is considered to be high. If dietary changes and exercise do not lead to a reduction, the NCEP recommends that cholesterol-lowering drugs be given serious consideration. Diet is the first line of defense, however, since cutting back on saturated fat will lead to a significant reduction in both total cholesterol and the LDL component for most people.[4] And if you are overweight, losing surplus pounds almost always results in a healthy reduction in LDL.

There are a number of different lipoprotein molecules circulating in the bloodstream, carrying fat and cholesterol to different locations in the body. In addition to LDL there are much smaller high-density molecules that contain a larger ratio of protein to lipid in their structure. High-density-lipoprotein (HDL) molecules appear to act as scavengers, bringing excess cholesterol back to the liver for reuse in the making of bile acid. Research consistently shows that a high ratio of HDL to LDL tends to lower the risk of heart disease. For example, a person having a total cholesterol of 200 ml/dl with an HDL count of 60 ml/dl would be at considerably less risk than a person with the same total cholesterol but an HDL count of only 30 ml/dl. Anything below an HDL of 35 ml/dl is considered risky.

But is your cholesterol level all that important?

There is no question that, in most cases, cutting saturated fat will result in a lowering of total cholesterol and the LDL component. But researchers have been asking themselves why people with cholesterol levels as high as 250 ml/dl in other parts of the world, such as in Mediterranean countries, have only half (or less) the risk of dying from heart disease as an American with a relatively "safe" cholesterol level of 190 ml/dl. Is there something in their diets that protects them in spite of having a cholesterol level that would clearly place them in the high-risk category in the United States?

The answer will become clear in a moment, after I explain how some of the processes involved in heart disease and cancer are similar.

---

[4]Whereas a 1 percent decrease in saturated-fat calories leads to an average decrease in total cholesterol of 2 ml/dl, it takes about a 100-milligram decrease in dietary cholesterol to achieve the same result. Only about 1 in 3 persons actually experiences any change in cholesterol level with a change in consumption of dietary cholesterol, but, while the amount will vary, almost all persons experience a reduction in cholesterol level when they reduce saturated fat in their diets.

THE CANCER CONNECTION

While total cholesterol and the LDL and HDL components may be rough markers for an increased risk of cardiovascular disease, research in the last couple of years suggests that it's not ordinary LDL that poses the real hazard. An elevated LDL component in your total cholesterol may prove to be of relatively little danger *unless your LDL cholesterol is being damaged by oxidation. In other words, the same process that can damage cell membranes and DNA, and which can lead to cancer, can damage LDL molecules and lead to heart disease.*

Lipids anywhere in the body are prime targets for free radicals, and LDL molecules have a lipid content of about 75 percent (50 percent cholesterol, 25 percent phospholipids and triglycerides). When LDL molecules are oxidized by free radicals their chemical structure is altered, and studies show that only the altered form of LDL appears to be involved in the formation of plaque on arterial walls—that is, atherosclerosis. It works in the following way.

As altered LDL particles flow through the arteries they come in contact with the endothelium, which is the layer of single cells that lines arterial walls. In contrast with normal, harmless LDL, altered LDL has a chemical structure that damages the lining and an SOS goes out to the immune system to send repair cells to the site to get rid of the dangerous LDL molecules. Macrophages, which are a kind of scavenging white blood cell, arrive and they ingest the oxidized LDL. However, absorbing the oxidized LDL causes the macrophages to bloat up and become transformed into "foam cells." The foam cells lodge under the arterial lining, and build up over time to form the artery-clogging plaque.

Now I think we have an answer as to under what conditions a cholesterol level of 250 ml/dl can be *less* dangerous than one of 190 ml/dl. *It depends upon the degree to which the LDL is being damaged by oxidation.*

How to Prevent the Oxidation of LDL

The immune system has several lines of defense aimed at preventing the oxidation of LDL by free radicals. It produces a number of different antioxidant proteins that are carried in the bloodstream and which defuse the free radicals before they can do any damage. Uric acid, a waste product carried in the blood, is also a potent free-radical scavenger. However, a high LDL level and the presence of too many free radicals within the bloodstream may overwhelm the body's self-generated internal defenses.

Here is where your diet plays a very important, potentially decisive, frontline role with rearguard action.

Vitamin C circulating in the bloodstream is the *first* antioxidant that springs into action to defuse free radicals. The body apparently keeps its own defenses in reserve until vitamin C is depleted. Vitamin C binds with free radicals *before* they can attack LDL molecules. As vitamin C is depleted, the body's own antioxidants go to work. Then come vitamin E and various carotenoids, including beta-carotene and lycopene, which form yet another line of antioxidant defense. Vitamin E and the carotenoids are fat soluble and pass into the LDL molecule and circulate with it. Free radicals that are not defused by vitamin C and the body's own free-radical scavengers can be intercepted as they attack the LDL molecules and rendered harmless by resident vitamin E and the carotenoids.

While research has demonstrated that LDL can be protected from oxidation by the antioxidant activity of the vitamins and carotenoids I've just mentioned, experts feel there are many more compounds among the thousands of flavonoids and hundreds of carotenoids found in the fruits, vegetables, and wine that are consumed in Mediterranean regions which are involved in explaining why a cholesterol of 250 ml/dl in Italy and Greece is less dangerous than one of 190 ml/dl in the United States. Not only do these phytochemicals help prevent oxidation of LDL, they also help keep the blood from becoming too viscous and therefore more likely to clot. In addition to these factors, the relatively low intake of saturated fat and high intake of monounsaturated fat found in olive oil (which is also a good source of the antioxidant vitamin E) may play an important role.

The conclusion to be drawn is this: Blood cholesterol level is a risk factor—one among many—for atherosclerosis. In all countries studied, as cholesterol levels increase, so does the risk of cardiovascular disease. But a diet rich in plant foods can help prevent the transformation of LDL into its dangerous oxidized form.

What can this mean to you? If you have a cholesterol level as high as 250 ml/dl, you may be able to cut your risk to *only half the risk that's normally associated with cholesterol levels of only 190 ml/dl in the United States!* The Cancer Prevention Good Health Diet is designed to help you do this.

A Further Similarity between Heart Disease and Cancer

There is another aspect in the development of atherosclerosis that suggests additional similarities between the causes of heart disease and cancer. Certain chemicals that act as initiators in the carcinogenic process by damaging DNA in the lungs and elsewhere, such as are found in cigarette smoke, have also been discovered bound to damaged DNA in the smooth-muscle layer of the arteries in patients with atherosclerosis. It is possible that changes caused by these carcinogenic compounds may contribute to the attraction of oxidized LDL and to the growth of plaque that can ultimately close off one or more arteries and lead to a heart attack. Thus, abnormal growths are characteristic of both cancer and heart disease.

You Can Only Depend on Real Foods to Cut Your Risk of Cardiovascular Disease and Cancer

I have used vitamins such as C and E, and beta-carotene, simply to illustrate the process by which they may build your immunity against cancer and cardiovascular disease. These substances are relatively easy to extract from foods, and they have been extensively examined in animal research and at the cellular level in the laboratory. But, as I have said before, individual nutrients do not do their work all alone, in isolation from the rest of your diet. It may take an entire army of phytochemicals, working together, to maximize the strength of your body's complex immune system. In the next chapter I'll explain how to recruit that phytochemical army to put the block on cancer, as well as heart disease.

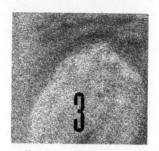

How to Build a Phytochemical Army to Fight Cancer and Heart Disease

The American Diet Is a Killer

Two out of three people alive today in the United States will ultimately die of cancer or heart disease. Experts estimate that about 60 percent of cancers in women and 40 percent in men are related to diet, as well as about 75 percent of the incidence of all heart disease. About a third of the incidence of both diseases is related to obesity.

Some of the foods we eat increase the likelihood of cancer and heart disease, while others can cut that likelihood at least by half. *Too much fat, too many calories, and too much red meat are the primary dietary culprits.* Herbicides, pesticides, and food additives are, when kept at legal limits, of relatively little danger in comparison.

How Too Much Fat Promotes Cancer

Too much fat is at the head of the danger list for cancer just as it is for heart disease. Among the many recent studies is one I'm looking at right now: it reports a laboratory experiment with mice indicating that the amount of fat in the typical American diet (about 40 percent of calories) can double the rate of growth in prostate cancer compared with the level recommended by just about all experts in the field (about 20 percent of calories),[1] which is the level I will help you achieve with the Cancer Prevention Good Health Diet.

There are a number of theories as to how fat might initiate and promote cancer.

1. Fat metabolism produces free radicals, which may damage cell membranes and DNA.
2. Fat increases the secretion of bile (an emulsifier) into the intestines, which can encourage the production of carcinogenic substances. In combination with a low-fiber diet, these carcinogens will remain for longer periods in the colon before being excreted and thus have more time to attack the cellular lining.
3. Fat helps promote the development of cancer by providing concentrated energy to cancer cells, which are dividing faster and need more energy than normal cells. In addition, too much fat may interfere with the command mechanism which tells cells to stop dividing.
4. Too much fat can alter the production of various hormones that are associated with cancer promotion—for example, in breast as well as prostate cancer.

Saturated fats are as significant in the cause of cancer as they are in heart disease. Studies show they increase the risk of colon, breast, prostate, ovarian, uterine, and skin cancers. In contrast with heart disease, however, where *polyunsaturated fat* (found mainly in vegetable oils other than olive, canola, and peanut) does not appear to elevate total cholesterol, too much polyunsaturated fat may be even more important than saturated fat as a risk factor for cancer. That's because there are more places in a polyunsaturated fat molecule where free radicals can attack the structure and find an electron mate. This, of course, damages the target molecule. Cellular membranes normally contain a large proportion of polyunsaturated fat, but since the chemical structure of fat in our body cells reflects the nature of the fats in our diet, some experts believe that a diet too high in polyunsaturated fat will add even more to our cellular membranes and make them more susceptible to free-radical attacks.

Monounsaturated fats, found predominantly in olive, canola, and

---

[1]As always, the researchers qualified their findings by pointing out that positive proof with respect to human prostate cancer requires clinical trials, where the diets of human subjects are controlled at the different levels of fat intake over long periods of time. "Proof-positive" research of this kind can take 25 years or more. If you are a male, can you afford to wait for the completion of human clinical trials?

peanut oils, are considered to be the least dangerous. As I have pointed out, in cultures where olive oil is the major source of fat in the diet (it also holds true for peanut oil), cardiovascular disease is less prevalent than in cultures where other fats are consumed in relatively larger quantities.

Too many calories in the diet aid the growth of cancer by providing an excess of energy that's put to use by the rapidly multiplying cancer cells. Along with too much fat of any kind, consuming too many calories is associated with obesity. While most people are aware of the connection between obesity and heart disease, they are not as aware that being overweight is also associated with a greater risk for colon and rectal cancer in men and a greater risk for cancer of the gallbladder, breast, cervix, endometrium, and ovary for women.

Is It Time to Cut Your Consumption of Red Meat?

I really can't pull punches here and do you the real service I intend. If you eat meat every day, or even just a few times a week, YES, IT'S TIME.

Although the underlying causes are not very well understood, more and more studies are suggesting an important connection between red meat and cancer. The consumption of red meat is frequently associated with a higher rate of cancer in epidemiological studies comparing the diets of different populations. Diets containing large quantities of red meat are high in protein, and a high-protein diet is a proven cancer risk in animal studies. A diet high in red meat is also usually associated with high fat and little fiber, and the three factors—high protein, high fat, and low fiber—may reinforce one another's dangerous effects. In addition, animal tissues, especially fat cells, concentrate the storage of toxins found in food, including pesticides and herbicides, to a far greater extent than is originally contained in the grains and other plant foods they have eaten. And, in my opinion, questions have not been satisfactorily answered about the safety, for human consumption, of meat and animal products that have been heavily treated with antibiotics and hormones.

An ongoing study being conducted at the School of Public Health at Harvard University, in which the diet and health of more than 88,000 nurses are being followed, found a clear relationship between the consumption of red meat—beef, lamb, and pork—and colon cancer. In a 1990 report, those who ate red meat daily were found to be two to three times more likely to develop the disease than those who ate red meat less than once a month. Since then, a number of other studies have appeared to support these findings.

These findings merit some additional comment, since representatives of the meat industry continually contest them and occasionally a study showing little relationship between fat or meat consumption and cancer is reported. Because they conflict with the mass of prior evidence, the results of this one contradictory study are widely disseminated in the media. The findings are almost always presented in "sound-bite" form, without adequate detail and objective scientific commentary from other experts. Perhaps you remember the hullabaloo over the one study that showed little impact of oat bran in the reduction of total cholesterol. This study made headlines and resulted in a drastic, and unfortunate, reduction in the consumption of oat bran and other oat products. What the media failed to note, and the researchers evidently failed to emphasize adequately, was that the subjects in the study already had low cholesterol levels. Their levels ranged between 180 and 190 ml/dl, which is already below the borderline range of 200–239 ml/dl and leaves little room for further decreases. Before and since that time, there have been *many* studies showing that oat bran and other foods containing soluble fiber help reduce *high* cholesterol levels.

In a similar vein, a recent study found no relationship between amount of fat in the diet and breast cancer. However, the women in the "low-fat" group were still consuming more than 30 percent of their calories in fat, which is well above the 20 percent level that most cancer experts suggest, and at which you will quite naturally arrive when you follow the Cancer Prevention Good Health Diet.

Proper Diet Can Protect You from Cancer

Over 200 studies have examined the relationship of diet to cancer in various countries and cultures. When data from these studies are combined, with people divided in quartiles according to their consumption of plant foods, *those in the highest quartile are between two and three times less likely to develop cancers of almost all varieties than those in the lowest quartile.*

Plant foods are protective foods.

The average American diet, high in fat, calories, and red meat, and with its low content of plant foods, is among the most deadly diets in the world. Only 9 percent of the U.S. population eat the *minimum* recommended number of servings of fruit and vegetables each day, almost half eat no fruit at all on a given day, and 1 out of 4 eat no vegetables![2]

[2]The American Cancer Society and other professional health organizations recommend a daily intake of from 5 to 9 servings of fruits and vegetables, combined.

It's not by chance that we have such a high rate of cancer and heart disease.

Enter Phytochemicals

Because the protective effect of plant foods is so consistent across all populations, and because certain foods (such as broccoli, cauliflower, brussels sprouts, cabbage, and other cruciferous vegetables; garlic and onions; and soybeans and other legumes) keep popping up in the diets of the people least likely to develop heart disease or cancer, scientists have become more and more curious about just what phytochemicals in the many different kinds of plant foods might be responsible.

Over a dozen different classes of phytochemicals and individual compounds, as well as some of the better-known vitamins and minerals, are receiving intensive study. The names of the vitamins are familiar (A, C, E, and folate, also called folic acid), as are the minerals (calcium and selenium). But, except perhaps for the carotenoids, the chemical names of the different phytochemicals are hardly household words. They include indoles, isoflavones, isothiocyanates, lignans, polyacetylene, protease inhibitors, quinones, saponins, sterols, sulfur, terpenes, and triterpenoids. I'll give you a good deal more information about all of them in a moment.

Protective phytochemicals appear to act in one of two main ways. Either directly as antioxidants, or indirectly by boosting production or increasing the activity of various enzymes, (1) they *block* carcinogenic agents, detoxifying them or keeping them from reaching or penetrating cell bodies, thus preventing the *initiation* of the carcinogenic process, or (2) they may *suppress* the expression of malignant changes in cells that have already been exposed and damaged by carcinogens, thus preventing the *promotion* of the carcinogenic process.

Putting the Block on Cancer

Because it usually takes so many years for cancer to develop, the body has many opportunities for blocking or suppressing its development, some of which I have described previously. In brief, if not directly carcinogenic, a precarcinogenic agent is first transformed into that common electrophilic form (see Chapter 1) that can attack cellular walls or DNA. Direct, blocking opportunities for many different phytochemicals, and for the protective enzymes that can be activated and strengthened by various phytochemicals, occur at several points along this route: in the bloodstream, stomach, and intestines, at the cellular walls, and within the cells. The aim here is to neutralize and dispose of any of the chemical compounds that can penetrate cell walls and damage DNA, or to repair damaged DNA before the cell divides and replicates.

Here are some examples and brief explanations of how certain vitamins and phytochemicals carry out their *blocking* function and protect the body against the *initiation* of the carcinogenic process. Some of these examples are based on laboratory research in which foods containing the different nutrients or phytochemicals, or extracts from these foods, are fed to laboratory animals and are seen to prevent or limit the development of experimentally induced malignant tumors. In other cases, extracts are placed in cultures of living cancer cells, and are seen to inhibit or limit the growth of different lines of experimentally induced cancer. The results of this controlled laboratory research support and help to explain why people who eat the most plant foods have the least cancer in epidemiological studies comparing the diets of different populations.

1. Ascorbic acid (vitamin C) and the phenols, all found in many different fruits and vegetables, *inhibit the transformation of precarcinogenic substances to carcinogenic forms.* For example, they scavenge nitrite in the gut and prevent it from combining with amines and forming nitrosamines, which are potent carcinogenic compounds.
2. Fiber *inhibits the uptake of carcinogens* from the gut into the circulatory system by absorbing them and allowing for harmless excretion, thus preventing the body from exposure to carcinogenic substances.
3. A number of different phytochemicals *interfere with the metabolism and activation of carcinogenic compounds.* Indoles and dithiothiones (cruciferous vegetables), flavonoids (in many fruits, vegetables, and tea), and sulfur compounds (garlic and onions) stimulate enzymes that deactivate precarcinogenic compounds and prevent their transformation into a more dangerous form.
4. The sulfur compounds from garlic and onions, dithiothiones and isothiocyanates from cruciferous vegetables, certain phenols in berries, other fruits, and tea, plus several carotenoids, ascorbic acid, and vitamin E in many fruits and vegetables all have strong antioxidant activity and *scavenge and remove free radicals and other electrophilic molecules* before they can attack susceptible points in body tissues.
5. The same phenols (as in the previous example) in fruits and tea bind with and deactivate free radicals and other carcinogenic compounds

inside cell bodies. This activity provides *direct protection to the DNA* from attacks that might otherwise cause dangerous mutations.

6. Protease inhibitors,[3] found particularly in soybeans, *activate enzymes that repair damaged DNA.* They also *inhibit cell proliferation,* which gives the repair enzymes a longer time period in which to make repairs to possibly dangerous DNA mutations.

Suppressing the Growth of Cancer

Should the initiation of the carcinogenic process already have occurred, phytochemicals have several avenues through which they can *suppress* the process and inhibit the *promotion* of a precancerous cell to a malignant state. In this way, the cell may lie dormant for a lifetime. Should the cell begin to grow and divide, some of the compounds may stimulate enzymes that convert the cell to a noncancerous form.

Here are some examples:

1. Certain flavonoids (such as quercetin, found in many plant foods), vitamin E (vegetable oils, nuts, grains), protease inhibitors (soybeans), and certain fibers *reduce the growth and inhibit the proliferation* of initiated, precancerous cells in experimental animals that have been given doses of various carcinogens.
2. Some carotenoids (for example, beta-carotene, in many fruits and vegetables) and terpenes (such as D-limonene, in citrus fruits) may lead a precancerous cell to *differentiate into a nonmalignant form,* or may cause it to *age quickly and become inactive.*
3. Selenium and vitamin E, quercetin, beta-carotene and other carotenoids, and vitamin C are all natural *antioxidants* that scavenge electrophilic substances which are toxic to cells and which ordinarily encourage a rapid cellular turnover. This scavenging activity inhibits tumor promotion by reducing the turnover of precancerous cells and preventing the expression of their potential for rapid cell division.

These two cancer-preventive mechanisms, *blocking the initiation* of the process and *suppressing the promotion* of initiated cells, form the basis for my recommendations in the Cancer Prevention Good Health Diet. The goal of the Cancer Prevention Good Health Diet is to make sure you are consuming the broad array of phytochemical agents that can maximize

[3]Protease is an enzyme that breaks down protein and facilitates cell growth and cell division. Protease inhibitors slow the process, resulting in the beneficial effects noted here.

your immune system's ability to intercept and render harmless carcinogenic and precarcinogenic substances and that can bolster the body's defenses against the promotion of any malignancies.

How and Why Did This Marvelous System of Cellular Defenses Develop?

The extraordinary defense process I have just described, together with that component of the immune system that protects us against bacterial and viral attack, has evolved over many millions of years. It is a product of our relationship with our environment and our ability to adapt. It developed to protect our species from the dangers the body faces and it draws upon substances found in the foods we eat for its strength.

But why plant foods in particular? Why did plants develop so many thousands of different chemicals and why did they become so important to human beings?

Origins of Plant Immunity and Its Relationship to Human Immunity against Cancer and Heart Disease

Scientists theorize that plant life as we know it began about 3.5 billion years ago, when plants, then living in a world devoid of oxygen, began turning carbon dioxide, with the help of light from the sun, into oxygen. This process creates waste products in the form of those unstable forms of oxygen we have been talking about—that is, free radicals and other electrophilic molecules—which can damage plant cells and plant DNA in the same way they can damage animal and human cells. Plants obviously needed to develop a way of dealing with this danger, and they did, in the form of *antioxidant* compounds.

Many of the phytochemicals that we are concerned with are part of a plant's antioxidant system, and some of them are easily identified because they are brightly colored and give different plants their distinctive hues. In addition to protecting against oxidation, many of these phytochemical compounds evolved to help plants protect themselves against other dangers, including climatic stress such as floods, dry spells, and extremes of temperature, and especially against threats from viruses, insects, and other organisms that prey upon them. And, yes, from plant cancers! Just like humans, waste products of plant metabolism and attacks from environmental carcinogenic agents can result in malignant growths in plants.[4]

The evolution of the human race has, of course, been closely intertwined with both the dangers and protections our ancestors found in their environment. Humans were originally a gathering species, and we existed primarily on plant foods. As the human immune system developed to battle infections and protect cells against dangerous substances that might result in cancer-causing mutations, it drew upon plant compounds for the essential ingredients. The building blocks for the army of enzymes (which are protein substances) that work to block or suppress carcinogenic substances are the nutrients in our foods: proteins, vitamins, and minerals. Phytochemicals appear to boost the activity and maintain the strength of these enzymes. In addition, many of the phytochemicals are themselves strong antioxidants and act directly, deactivating free radicals and other electrophiles. Still others appear to interfere with the binding of hormones to cells, such as estrogen, which under certain conditions can stimulate the growth of a cancer.

Scientists are not yet completely certain how individual phytochemicals work in the human body. They can, however, see how the growth of cancer cells in cultures is blocked when extracts from plant foods that seem to protect against cancer in the human diet (soybeans, garlic, broccoli, tea, and many others) are added to these cultures. They can also see the end result in controlled studies using live animals: fewer cancers in experimental animals given these foods or extracts while exposed to carcinogenic substances, compared with control animals on a standard animal diet.

Putting the results of these laboratory studies together with the evidence gathered from examining the diets of people around the world has convinced all experts in the field that a diet high in plant foods can cut your risk of cancer at least in half.

Table 3.1 contains a list of protective phytochemicals together with foods known at the present time to contain them in significant quantities and the general mechanisms of action believed to be involved in the prevention of cancer. Because not all common foods, herbs, and spices have been studied, the list is certainly incomplete and sure to be expanded in the next few years. It's almost certain that, in addition to their vitamin and mineral content, many other foods, herbs, and spices will be found to contain phytochemicals that block or suppress the development of cancer.

Table 3.2 contains some in-depth botanical, biological, and chemical

---

[4]Perhaps very important in the development of defense mechanisms in plants is that they can't run away from predators—they had to develop chemical defenses to survive.

Table 3.1 THE PHYTOCHEMICAL ARMAMENTARIUM

Phytochemical	Foods	Physiological Activity
Carotenoids (includes carotenes)	Broccoli Cantalope Carrots Kale Pumpkin Spinach Squash Sweet potatoes Yams	Antioxidant; strengthen immune system; suppress and may reverse precancerous conditions
Catechins (tannins)	Berries Green and black teas	Antioxidant
Flavonoids	Bell peppers Berries Broccoli Cabbage Carrots Citrus fruits Cucumbers Eggplant Parsley Soybeans Soy products Squash Tomatoes Yams	Bind with and inhibit hormones that can encourage the growth of cancers; antioxidant
Indoles	Bok choy Broccoli Brussels sprouts Cabbage Cauliflower Collards Kale Kohlrabi Mustard greens Rutabaga Turnips	Inactivate estrogen, which fuels growth of breast cancer; stimulate protective enzymes, some of which block carcinogens, while others suppress tumor growth
Isoflavones	Beans Peanuts and other legumes Peas	Inactivate estrogen and block estrogen receptors; destroy enzymes produced by cancer genes

Table 3.1 THE PHYTOCHEMICAL ARMANENTARIUM (*continued*)

Phytochemical	Foods	Physiological Activity
Isothiocyanates	Cruciferous vegetables (see list under "Indoles") Horseradish Mustard Radishes	Stimulate protective enzymes, some of which block carcinogens, while others suppress tumor growth
Lignans	Flaxseed Walnuts Other nuts and seeds	Antioxidant; inactivate estrogen; block hormones that promote cancer
Liminoids	Citrus fruits	Stimulate protective enzymes
Lycopene	Red grapefruit Tomatoes	Antioxidant
Monoterpenes	Basil Broccoli Cabbage Caraway seeds Carrots Citrus fruits Cucumber Eggplant Mint Parsley Peppers Squash Tomatoes Yams	Antioxidant; stimulate protective enzymes
Omega-3 polyunsaturated fatty acids	Flaxseed Walnuts	Inactivate estrogen; block action of other cancer-promoting hormones
Phenolic acids	Berries Broccoli Cabbage Carrots Citrus fruits Eggplant Parsley Peppers Tomatoes Whole grains	Antioxidant; inhibit formation of nitrosamines; suppress acitvity of cancer-promoting enzymes

Table 3.1 THE PHYTOCHEMICAL ARMANENTARIUM (*continued*)

Phytochemical	Foods	Physiological Activity
Plant sterols	Broccoli Cabbage Cucumbers Eggplant Peppers Soybeans Soy products Squash Tomatoes Whole grains Yams	Encourage differentiation of precancerous cells to a noncancerous form
Polyacetylenes	Aniseed Caraway Carrots Celery Chervil Coriander Cumin Dill Fennel Parsley Parsnip	Suppress activity of cancer-promoting hormones; destroy benzo[a]pyrene (a potent carcinogen)
Protease inhibitors	Soybeans Soy products	Destroy enzymes that can cause cancer to spread
Quinones	Rosemary	Inhibit carcinogens and co-carcinogens that help activate carcinogens
Sulfur compounds	Garlic Leeks Onions Shallots	Inhibit carcinogens and suppress tumor development
Terpenes	Citrus fruits	Stimulate enzymes that block carcinogens
Triterpenes	Licorice root	Inactivate estrogen and other cancer-promoting hormones; slow proliferation of cancer cells

Table 3.2 NATURE'S CHEMOPROTECTIVE ARMY: FACTS AND DEFINITIONS

Carotenoids	There are some 600 different carotenoids divided primarily into two main groups: carotenes and xanthophylls. Carotenoids impart yellow, orange, or red colors to flowers (dandelions and marigolds), fruits (apricots, pumpkins, tomatoes, citrus fruits), and roots (carrots, sweet potatoes, yams). Many animals convert provitamin (source of vitamin) carotenes (there are about 50 of them) to vitamin A in their livers. To date, the most important one for human consumption appears to be beta-carotene, and it is during the conversion process that most experts believe we obtain its anticarcinogenic benefits. While beta-carotene is considered to be one of the most potent neutralizers of free radicals in the group, all the carotenes have antioxidant activity. Because studies using beta-carotene supplementation have yielded inconsistent results, some researchers are beginning to believe that it may require the presence of other constituents in food to work efficiently. They are also beginning to think that other carotenoids may ultimately prove to be the real cancer inhibitors and that the various carotenoids may have different and perhaps specific effects on different types of carcinogens and different kinds of tumors. Furthermore, many experts are beginning to think that beta-carotene, when found in relatively large amounts in the blood plasma, may simply be a good marker for the presence of the wide variety of anticarcinogenic substances that are being ingested by people who eat a large number of fruits and vegetables. Whatever the case may be, high levels of beta-carotene have been associated with lower risk of lung, breast, cervical, uterine, esophageal, stomach, colon, and mouth cancers. In addition, beta-carotene, or its associated carotenoids, may suppress cancers of the cervix and uterus after they have begun, and possibly reverse precancerous lesions in the mouth.
Catechins	Catechins, or tannins, are members of the class of plant structures called phenols. This class also includes the flavonoids (see below), to which tannins are similar in chemical structure. Like certain flavonoids, they have antioxidant activity, and extracts from tea (ellagic and tannic acids) have been shown to inhibit the activity of enzymes that promote cancer.
Flavonoids	There are about 4000 different flavonoids, including pigments called anthocyanins (which give plants orange and red to blue colors, and are responsible for purple and purple-reds in autumn leaves) and flavones (which are yellow and white). Flavonoids, which are a group of compounds in the phenol class (like tannins), are found in many fruits, vegetables, and wine (see Table 3.1). Many of them have antioxidant activity; some may act as blockers of carcinogens, while others may suppress malignant changes in

	cell processes. Flavonoids appear to bind with and inhibit the activity of hormones that promote cancer.
Indoles	Like isothiocyanates (see below), indoles are created as breakdown products when foods containing glucosinolates are chewed or cooked. There are about 80 different glucosinolates and they are prominent in cruciferous vegetables. Indoles appear to have a variety of different functions, including the inhibition of the cancer-forming potential of estrogen and the activation of carcinogen-blocking enzymes.
Isoflavones	A particular group of flavonoids found prominently in legumes, especially soybeans, isoflavones are antioxidants, and appear capable of both blocking and suppressing activity in helping to prevent breast and prostate cancers. These two forms of cancer are far less frequent in Asian women and men, for whom soybeans and soy products are dietary mainstays. Genistein, biochanin A, and daidzein are three forms of isoflavones that may inactivate enzymes produced by cancer genes, thereby inhibiting the growth and propagation of cancer cells.
Isothiocyanates	Like indoles, isothiocyanates are breakdown products of glucosinolates when foods containing these compounds are chewed or cooked. Isothiocyanates are responsible for the slightly acrid and bitter "bite" associated with cruciferous vegetables such as broccoli, cauliflower, and other foods in the cabbage family. These compounds appear to activate both carcinogen-blocking and tumor-growth-suppressing enzymes.
Lignans	Lignans are found in small amounts in many different plant fibers. They are a mixture of compounds in the same class of plant chemicals called phenolics that are found in flavonoids and quinones, and like other phenolics, they have antioxidant properties. So far, they have been found to be especially abundant in linseed (flaxseed) and walnuts, and they may both block and suppress carcinogenic changes. Studies have shown specific blocking of hormones such as estrogen and prostaglandins that can promote the spread of cancer. Although not yet tested, many scientists believe that nuts and seeds in general, because they are very stable living organisms, will prove to be strong antioxidants and may contain the greatest quantities of these cancer-preventive compounds.
Liminoids	There are about 100 different liminoids and they belong to the class of phytochemicals called terpenes (or terpenoids, interchangeably, although the latter term is more precisely reserved for the oxygenated form). This large class of phytochemicals contains about 7500 different compounds, including, among others with anticar-

cinogenic activity, monoterpenes, diterpenes, triterpenes, and carotenoids (which are tetraterpenes; see terpenes, below). Liminoids are found in citrus fruits and contribute to their bitter taste. They stimulate protective enzymes.

Lycopene   A specific carotenoid that gives the color red to tomatoes and red grapefruit. Like other carotenoids, it is an antioxidant.

Monoterpenes   Members of the terpene group, monoterpenes number about 1000 and give many different vegetables, fruits, and herbs their pleasant smells. They have some antioxidant activity and have also been shown to activate protective enzymes.

Omega-3 polyunsaturated fatty acids   Found alongside lignans in flaxseed and walnuts, omega-3 fatty acids inhibit hormones such as estrogen and prostaglandins, which promote the growth of certain cancers. These are the same fatty acids that have a protective role in cardiovascular disease.

Phenolic acids   These acids belong in the same group of phenolics as flavonoids and quinones, and like flavonoids, they have antioxidant activity. They also inhibit the creation of nitrosamines, compounds that are formed through a combination of nitrites and amines during the digestive process. Nitrites and amines are found naturally in many foods, and nitrites are added to processed meats to inhibit rancidity and prevent the growth of bacteria. Nitrosamines can be dangerous in large quantities, but the amount formed as a consequence of the typical American diet is not thought to be harmful. A cigarette smoker inhales 100 times the amount of nitrosamines that can result from a meal containing a serving of bacon or other processed meat.

Plant sterols   Sterols are a type of lipid found in many forms in both plants and animals. In the human body, bile acids and sex and adrenal hormones are sterols, as is cholesterol, which constitutes an essential part of cell membranes. In humans, plant sterols act as precursors to vitamin D and they may play a role in the differentiation of cancer cells during replication, changing their characteristics and suppressing further growth.

Polyacetylenes   There are about 650 different polyacetylenes and they occur in many important foods, herbs, spices, and flavorings, including dill, chervil, celery, caraway, coriander, cumin, carrots, fennel, parsley, parsnip, and aniseed among others. Certain polyacetylenes (one has been found in parsley) may suppress the activity of cancer-promoting hormones, while others may help destroy benzo[a]-pyrene, a potent carcinogen created during the grilling of meat, when fat hits the fire. In addition to their potential as anticarcinogens, polyacetylenes are antimicrobial and herbs containing polyacetylenes have been used in folk medicine for hundreds of years.

Table 3.2 NATURE'S CHEMOPROTECTIVE ARMY: FACTS AND DEFINITIONS (*continued*)

Protease inhibitors	Proteases (for example, trypsin and chymotrypsin) are enzymes that break down (hydrolyze) protein into smaller molecules during the digestive process. While limiting their action, protease inhibitors also limit other activities, such as the rate of cell division. By slowing the rate at which a cell will divide, more time is given to the enzymes that facilitate the repair of damaged DNA. It is also possible that protease inhibitors play a more direct role by increasing the activity of the repair enzymes themselves, as well as giving them more time to do their work. These two activities may prevent the conversion of normal cells to malignant cells in the early stages of cancer development. Soybeans and soy products are rich sources of these inhibitors, and cereals to a lesser extent. Protease inhibitors have been shown to limit the development of colon, lung, mouth, liver, and esophageal cancers in animals.
Quinones	There are about 800 different quinones, a subgroup of phenolics. Some of them impart a red or yellow color to parts of plants. Quinones are found in certain herbs, especially rosemary, and they appear to inhibit carcinogens and co-carcinogens (substances that facilitate carcinogenic activity).
Sulfur compounds	Sulfur compounds are found in plants from the genus *Allium*, which includes garlic, onions, leeks, and shallots. Diallyl disulfide appears to be the most effective of these compounds (allylic sulfides) in inhibiting carcinogens and suppressing the enzymes that cause cancers to spread. Garlic is the richest of the group in its diallyl disulfide content. Isothiocyanates formed during the breakdown of cruciferous vegetables may also contain sulfur, which may facilitate their cancer-protective activity.
Terpenes	Also known as isoprenoids, terpenes are a large group of plant chemicals from which terpenoids are formed by the addition of oxygen, with which they readily combine, and which gives them their important antioxidant capability. Numbering in the thousands, they assume different forms which differ in the degree of molecular complexity, such as monoterpenes, diterpenes, and triterpenes. Monoterpenes impart a pleasant smell, while the more complex terpenes are often bitter. Vitamin A is a diterpene, while carotenoids such as beta-carotene are tetraterpenes. Tetraterpene molecules are twice the size of diterpenes, so when a beta-carotene molecule is split during the process by which the body makes vitamin A, the antioxidant activity may be at its height. In addition to antioxidant activity, the particular terpenes found in citrus fruits stimulate enzymes that block carcinogens.
Triterpenes	Members of the terpene class of phytochemicals, those found in licorice limit the activity of hormones that promote cancer, such as

How to Build a Phytochemical Army to Fight Cancer and Heart Disease

33

estrogen and prostaglandins, and slow the rate at which cancer cells divide and replicate. Oil of anise (which does not contain these triterpenes) has a licorice flavor, and it is normally used to give the flavor of licorice in the United States because true licorice from the leguminous plant *Glycyrrhiza glabra* can be toxic when consumed regularly in what some people might consider modest amounts (for example, as little as 3 ounces of licorice twists, made with true licorice, per day over time; see Chapter 8 for a general discussion of the toxicity issue with respect to phytochemicals and my comment on phytochemical supplementation in the epilogue). True licorice root can be found in health-food stores and is present, in small amounts, in certain herb teas (check the labels and, if you choose to use them, be moderate in your consumption).

information on the different classes of phytochemicals plus some additional information on how they contribute to our health.

Traditional Nutrients and the Prevention of Disease

While my primary emphasis here is on helping you to design a diet that includes the protective phytochemicals I've been describing, you must still include the traditional vitamins and minerals ("nutrients") for the essential roles they play in maintaining your health throughout your life. At the present time, certain distinctions are made between nutrients and phytochemicals that may appear rather confusing. I hope the following discussion will help clear that up.

WHY ARE VITAMINS AND CERTAIN MINERALS CALLED "NUTRIENTS"?

Vitamins and certain minerals are called nutrients because they provide the nourishment that's *essential* to human growth and the prevention of certain diseases. The word *vitamin* is a combination of the terms *vita,* meaning "life," and *amine,* which is a scientific term given to a particular category of chemical compounds. While they do not provide energy and are needed in only minute quantities by the human body, vitamins perform essential functions as coenzymes or precursors to coenzymes. In one way or another, virtually all metabolic processes depend on vitamins and certain minerals, and when these are lacking in the diet, or they cannot be manufactured in the human body from other substances, we sicken and ultimately die. In other words, life depends on them.

Vitamin C is a classic and dramatic example of what is meant by a nutrient, and of the disease-prevention process through which the essential nature of a nutrient was discovered during the last few hundred years.

Two hundred and fifty years ago, a British sailor on a long ocean voyage had barely a fifty-fifty chance of returning home alive. The reason was not that he might be killed by pirates or die in a storm, but that he would die of the dread disease scurvy. Only sailors on short voyages— for example, in the Mediterranean—escaped it. Looking for an explanation, James Lind, a British physician, thought it might lie in the kind of food provided, because ship cooks used up the fresh fruit and vegetables first, and, on long ocean voyages, the men had to survive on meat and cereals.

In 1747 he devised an experiment in which six different groups of sailors who were suffering from scurvy received a different supplemental ration: either cider, vinegar, sulfuric acid, seawater, oranges and lemons, or a purgative mixed with spices. Only those receiving the citrus fruits quickly recovered.

No one knew for sure why these men recovered, and it took another 50 years before the British navy required that all voyaging sailors receive a daily ration of lime juice (from which time they became known as "limeys"). The unknown substance in limes and other foods that prevented (or cured) scurvy was called the antiscorbutic factor. It was not until almost 200 years later that the actual chemical compound that prevented scurvy was isolated, and named ascorbic acid. Ascorbic acid is one of the two active forms of vitamin C, and the form whose chemical structure also allows it to play its very important role as an antioxidant in the human body.[5]

Nutrients such as vitamin C, certain other vitamins, and certain minerals play dual roles. They support human growth and prevent deficiency diseases (such as scurvy) that can occur at any time of life if and when these nutrients are absent from the diet. But they are also active throughout life in the prevention of degenerative diseases whose frequency begins to increase with age, such as cancer and heart disease.

[5]Dehydroascorbic acid is the second, oxidized form of vitamin C. As ascorbic acid, vitamin C has two hydrogen atoms that can be donated to electron-hungry free radicals. By offering itself for oxidation, ascorbic acid prevents the oxidation and possible subsequent damage of other cellular components. Dehydroascorbic acid can still function as a vitamin, but not as an antioxidant.

ARE PHYTOCHEMICALS ALSO NUTRIENTS?

The phytochemicals that are the focus of the Cancer Prevention Good Health Diet and which appear to play key roles in the prevention of cancer and heart disease are not classified as nutrients at the present time. They are sometimes called "secondary plant compounds." As I mentioned earlier, scientists don't know exactly how individual phytochemicals work and they don't know if the lack of any single phytochemical or single class of phytochemicals invariably leads to illness or death, as it does with vitamins and certain minerals. Our state of knowledge is, in some respects, like that of the physicians who knew that citrus fruits prevented or cured scurvy without knowing exactly why for almost 200 years. Without knowing exactly why, we, today, know that people who eat the greatest amount of plant foods have half or less the rate of cancer compared with those who eat the least. And we are discovering that the different phytochemicals in the various classes act in different ways and work together. It may be many years before as much knowledge is available about the role of phytochemicals in human health as we now have with respect to vitamins and minerals. Rather than wait, I think the best advice is simply to eat a wide variety of plant foods, with fruits and vegetables of various colors every day.

Key Vitamins and Minerals that May Help Protect Against Cancer and Heart Disease

BETA-CAROTENE/VITAMIN A

Plants do not contain any pre-formed vitamin A. They contain a precursor called beta-carotene, which is a carotenoid pigment that gives plants their yellow/orange color. Sometimes the presence of beta-carotene is hidden by a cloak of chlorophyll, which colors the plant green. Vitamin A is formed when beta-carotene, as well as a number of other carotenoids, is broken down in the intestines and liver. Only animals and animal products contain pre-formed vitamin A.

Vitamin A, in whatever way it is obtained, has several major roles in the human body. In addition to promoting vision, maintaining the health of skin and other epithelial tissues, and promoting growth and the remodeling of our bones as they grow throughout our youth, vitamin A has long been known to play an important part in maintaining the strength of the immune system. In fact, as far back as the 1920s, vitamin A became known as the "anti-infective" vitamin because its presence seemed to

MY TOP 20 SOURCES OF BETA-CAROTENE[a]

Pumpkin	Bok choy
Sweet potato	Mustard greens
Carrot	Collard greens
Spinach	Parsley
Butternut squash	Apricots
Winter squash	Broccoli
Cantaloupe	Watermelon
Mango	Asparagus
Turnip greens	Romaine lettuce
Papaya	Tomato (and tomato juice)[b]

[a]While foods in my Top 20 lists are in order of richness in the specific nutrient, those farther down on the list may be highest in other protective nutrients and phytochemicals. Therefore, it's a good idea to think in terms of variety, and not limit yourself to those that happen to contain a large amount of any single nutrient or phytochemical compound. I have intentionally left red meat off any list in which it might rank among the top 20 in absolute content of that nutrient because of other considerations that I have discussed in the main text. My lists contain commonly used foods that are easy to find in supermarkets, and the amount of the nutrient was determined per average serving. Rare or exotic foods have been omitted.

[b]In this and the following lists, the nutrient is more concentrated in the form outside the parentheses, but that within the parentheses is also a good to excellent source.

lower the risk and severity of a number of infections in children. Recent studies show that it reduces the morbidity of children born to HIV-infected mothers.

Most research suggests, however, that protection from cancer may be due to the presence of beta-carotene and possibly the other carotenoids in the diet, and not pre-formed vitamin A. Various studies show that persons eating a diet high in plant foods containing beta-carotene, or who have high levels of beta-carotene in their blood, have far lower rates of various cancers, including cancers of the lung, breast, cervix, uterus, esophagus, stomach, colon, and mouth. Some experts believe it is not beta-carotene alone that provides the protection, but that beta-carotene is simply a marker for the presence of a large variety of protective carotenoids and other phytochemicals that will be present in the body when one eats a diet high in plant foods. The likelihood that this is the case will become evident when you compare the foods in the following list of best sources of beta-carotene with the list of foods high in various protective phytochemicals in Table 3.1. There is a tremendous amount of overlap. Foods high in beta-carotene carry with them an arsenal of other chemoprotective compounds.

VITAMIN C

Vitamin C plays an important role as a coenzyme in the conversion of amino acids to the protein forms needed to build various body tissues, and it has been known as an immune system booster for many years. But it is in its role as an antioxidant that it may protect against cancer and heart disease. In a sense, vitamin C sacrifices its own life, that is, its structure, by donating a couple of electrons to electrophilic compounds that might otherwise steal electrons from body cells or attack LDL molecules in the bloodstream. In this way, it detoxifies potential carcinogens present in cigarette smoke, industrial pollutants, automobile exhaust, and pesticides. If you are exposed to these carcinogenic substances, I'd recommend double servings of foods rich in vitamin C!

More than 30 studies have shown that persons who consume a diet rich in vitamin C foods have a reduced risk of many different cancers, including those of the lung, esophagus, larynx, mouth, pancreas, rectum, breast, cervix, and pancreas.

VITAMIN E

Vitamin E is a fat-soluble vitamin that acts as one of the body's most potent antioxidants. Like vitamin C, it protects the body against oxidation by sacrificing itself. Its action complements that of vitamin C, which is a water-soluble vitamin. While vitamin C protects against carcinogens in the watery parts of cells and in blood plasma, vitamin E protects against carcinogens that might attack lipid parts of cells, such as the cell membranes or molecules of LDL. It is especially potent as a protector of cellular membranes, where it prevents free-radical attacks that result in the oxidation

---

MY TOP 20 SOURCES OF VITAMIN C

Papaya	Parsley
Orange juice (and oranges)	Asparagus
Broccoli	Watermelon
Cantaloupe	Tomato juice (and tomato)
Brussels sprouts	Bok choy
Grapefruit juice (and grapefruit)	Turnip greens
Strawberries	Butternut squash
Cauliflower	Mustard greens
Green bell pepper	Cabbage
Mango	Baked potato

MY TOP 20 SOURCES OF VITAMIN E

Wheat-germ oil	Canola oil
Sunflower seeds, dry	Soybean oil
Sweet potato	Peanut oil (and peanuts)
Sunflower-seed oil	Olive oil
Almond oil	Brazil nuts
Cottonseed oil	Hazelnuts
Safflower oil	Cashews
Peanut butter, chunky	Salmon
Shrimp (boiled)	Avocado
Corn oil	Sole/flounder

of unsaturated fatty acids (called "lipid peroxidation"). Without vitamin E to intercede, cell structures would be damaged and unable to function in their normal manner. Vitamin E also protects both red and white blood cells and thus helps maintain our immune defenses.

Vitamin E may be especially important for people who live where the air is highly polluted by ozone and automobile or industrial fumes. It protects not only cells in the lung tissue from these pollutants, but also the red and white blood cells that flow through the lungs and which might be adversely affected by pollutants in the air.

Eating foods rich in vitamin E has been shown to protect against lung, breast, stomach, cervical, pancreatic, and urinary-tract cancers.

Vitamin E is widespread in foods, but, as a fat-soluble vitamin, it is not found in particularly large amounts in plant foods except in their oils, and in nuts and seeds. Because oils, nuts, and seeds contain a large proportion of polyunsaturated fatty acids, it seems as though Mother Nature was wise to include this potent antioxidant, vitamin E, along with the fat!

While not in sufficient quantity to rank them in the top 20 sources (because they contain so little fat), additional good sources of vitamin E include green leafy vegetables, whole-grain products, and dried beans. Fortified cereals are also good sources.

OTHER NUTRIENTS WITH PROTECTIVE ACTION

Folate, also known as folic acid, plays a key role in the regulation of cell division, protein synthesis, and prevention of birth defects. Studies show a protective role in colon cancer and, most recently, a possibly critical role in the prevention of heart disease. Vegetables and legumes are your best sources.

Calcium, the most abundant mineral in the human body, is also one of the most important for its function as the principal mineral in bones and teeth, and for its role in the transmission of nerve impulses, regulation of muscle contractions, blood clotting, blood pressure, and immune defenses. New research suggests that calcium may protect against colon cancer by limiting potentially dangerous cell growths and binding potential carcinogens to fatty acids that will be excreted.

Selenium is a mineral that is needed in only the tiniest amounts (less than 0.1 milligram per day), but which plays an important role as part of a very important antioxidant enzyme called *glutathione peroxidase.* This enzyme is produced by the human body to prevent the oxidation of fatty acids, and it is known to work together with vitamin E to protect the fatty parts of body cells. There is also some evidence that it works in collaboration with other phytochemicals, beta-carotene, and vitamin C. That is, it can't do its job without its helpers.

While animal products are reliable sources of selenium because it is associated with the protein parts of foods, it is also found in plant foods grown in selenium-rich soils. The presence of selenium in the soil may also enhance the cancer-inhibiting power of other phytochemicals found in foods (such as garlic) that are grown in that soil. There is considerable ongoing research about this possibility. In general, seafood and grains are to be preferred as sources of selenium, compared with meat.

Vitamin D is different from other essential nutrients in that the body can synthesize it, with the help of sunlight, from a cholesterol-like substance in our skin. Exposing hands, face, and arms to sunlight for about 10 to 15 minutes a few times a week seems to supply all bodily needs in fair-skinned people, while in dark-skinned people it may take about an hour.

Vitamin D is not present naturally in significant amounts in food, other than in egg yolks, liver, and fatty fish. Therefore, people restricted from going outdoors or who live in cloudy or smoggy areas should include in their diets foods such as milk and cereals that are fortified with vitamin D.

In recent years, researchers have found that vitamin D acts like a hormone, crossing cellular walls in many different body tissues from the brain to the bones to the kidneys, to promote a great variety of cellular functions, including regulation of the immune system and the secretion of insulin. Some studies show that vitamin D may help protect against colon cancer, and a recent study has shown that it may facilitate the action of insulin and help regulate blood sugar, and also help prevent high blood pressure.

Your Most Powerful Cancer Fighting Antioxidant Foods

While phytochemicals work in several different ways to protect against cancer and heart disease, certain ones have greater antioxidant activity than others. That is, they have a greater capacity to reduce the activity of cell and DNA damaging free radicals. Those with especially high antioxidant potential are called high-ORAC (oxygen radical absorbance capacity) phytochemicals. In general, it's the carotenoids and flavonoids that provide the greatest ORAC. As you know from our previous discussion, these particular phytochemicals are actually pigments, some of which give foods their brilliant or deep colors.

Scientists have recently devised a method for measuring the ORAC in human blood after different foods have been consumed. Various fruits and vegetables, in the order of their cancer fighting ORAC, include:

Prunes	Broccoli
Raisins	Beets
Blueberries	Red bell peppers
Strawberries	Oranges
Raspberries	Red grapes
Plums	Cherries
Kale	Yellow corn
Spinach	Eggplant
Brussels sprouts	Carrots

Fruit and vegetable juices tend also to contain significant amounts of high-ORAC phytochemicals, and the protective substances are even somewhat more concentrated in dried fruits than in fresh. As you can see from the above list, high-ORAC foods are richly colored, so make it a point to include a variety of them in your daily diet, and color yourself healthy!

I've tried in this chapter to give you a convincing rationale for cutting down on things in your diet that might be dangerous to your health—fat, calories, and red meat—and increasing those things that can contribute to a happier, healthier, and longer life—fruits, vegetables, and grains. Now I'd like to show you how to do it in a way that you will come to enjoy as much as, maybe even more than, your present diet.

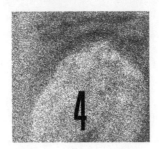

The Cancer Prevention Good Health Diet

PART 1: GENERAL GUIDELINES

It's one thing to be handed a bunch of good dietary advice. It's quite another to be shown how to follow that advice, easily and enjoyably.

My primary goal in this book is to show you not only what you need to do on a daily basis, but *how* to do it. I know that there is very little likelihood you will stick with a diet that promises you a healthier, happier life 20, 30, or 40 years down the road if you have to feel miserable and inconvenienced today and every other day in order to get there.

I've promised: no deprivation. As you begin to experiment with my recipes and my suggestions about how to prepare a tasty, healthful diet, I think you will find that I fulfill that promise. In contrast with many diet books written by prominent health professionals, who often hire out the development of recipes and the design of menus, every one of the recipes in this book has been prepared by me and my wife, often in several versions, and tested among friends and professional colleagues until we all agreed that they taste good enough to take their place as a permanent part of a person's diet. A simple "That's okay" didn't cut it. They all had to be good enough to make us look forward to having them again and again.

But how about feeling good and convenience?

My 3-step approach to helping you make a transition to a more healthful way of eating is so graduated and easy, you will never feel that any sacrifice is involved. I think one of the most serious mistakes you might make when you're interested in improving your diet is to try to do too much in too little time. You are not "going on a diet" with all changes due in place tomorrow. That's self-defeating, and besides, that drastic a change might make you feel temporarily uncomfortable.

How Good Is Your Present Diet?

Before you begin to study the Cancer Prevention Good Health guidelines and develop a plan of action, take time to answer the questions in the following quiz, just to see where you stand today in relation to our ultimate goals. Recall what you have eaten so far today, and think back over what you have eaten during the last couple of days.[1]

1. Do you eat 6 to 11 servings of grain foods each day (bread, cereal, rice, and pasta included)?
2. Are half or more of these servings from whole grains or high-fiber cereals (whole-wheat pasta, whole-grain breads, brown rice, oatmeal)?
3. Do you eat 5 to 9 servings of fruits and vegetables (combined) each day?
4. Does this include a deep-green leafy vegetable every day?
5. Do you eat 3 or more different-colored fruits and vegetables, including those with red and yellow/orange colorations or shades of these colors, every day?
6. Do you eat cruciferous vegetables several times a week, such as broccoli, cauliflower, cabbage, kale, collards, or other members of the cabbage family?
7. Do you include liberal amounts of garlic, onions, leeks, or shallots in your diet?
8. Do you include among your fruits 1 or 2 servings of a citrus fruit each day?
9. If and when you eat red meat, do you eat only the leanest cuts?
10. Do you eat more fish, poultry, and legumes than you do red meat?
11. Do you use primarily low-fat dairy products?
12. If you use alcohol, do you limit consumption to no more than 1 (women) or 2 (men) drinks a day?

Although this short quiz is not meant to cover the entire nutritional ballpark, only a "yes" answer to *all* these questions means that you are safely on the path to achieving the maximum immunity that diet can give you

---

[1]It would be more accurate to write everything down for a few days, but most people will get a pretty good idea from this general recall approach, and most people don't care to take the time to do this kind of an eating record.

against cancer, heart disease, stroke, adult-onset diabetes, and other de-generative illnesses. Fewer than 1 in 10 persons in the United States can give a positive answer to all these questions.

"Yes" answers to the above quiz embody the final, most important, *practical, day-by-day* objectives of the Cancer Prevention Good Health Diet. A diet based on "yes" answers would include the important immunity-enhancing phytochemicals that we've been talking about, and it would minimize the dangerous fats, surplus calories, and red meat.

But if you have been eating the typical American diet, *these objectives are not to be reached tomorrow, in one giant step.* A change that sudden might make you very uncomfortable because of the increase in fiber content. And, if you are accustomed to more meat and fat, attempting to delete so many of your favorite foods in one fell swoop, before you have had a chance to develop new taste preferences in a natural way, would certainly make you feel deprived and probably irritable!

Goals and Guidelines

In this chapter I want to provide you with the general guidelines for the Cancer Prevention Good Health Diet, including the 3-step plan. I think this simple plan makes improving your diet easier and more interesting than any other way of which I am aware. In the next chapter I will give you a suggested sequence for trying various recipes that I think will demonstrate to you that eating in the most healthful way tastes just as good as, maybe even better than, your present diet. I will also give you some suggested meal plans and daily menus to serve as models to aim for over the next couple of months. I think you will discover some additional benefits as you do this. For example, if you often feel uncomfortable after eating, or lacking in energy at certain times during the day, I think you will find yourself grad-ually beginning to feel better than you have ever felt before.

If you follow my suggestions in this chapter and in the following one, the changes we're aiming for will take place so easily you will hardly be aware that they are happening. One day you may stop to reflect and re-alize that you have made a completely painless transition to a healthful diet, without any particular effort and with no sacrifice at all!

THE 3-STEP PLAN

The plan is to go one recipe, one meal, one day at a time, until step by step you reach the final goal. There is no prescription for an entirely new meal plan to be put into practice tomorrow. I think you will be surprised at how easy it is to go just one recipe at a time. Each week I want you to try 2 or 3 different recipes, based primarily on plant foods, picked from the great number in Chapter 7. You can follow my suggested sequence of recipes, or pick your own after checking them all out. Either way, within a month or two, you will be introduced to a variety of different foods and some delicious methods of preparation.

SOME SPECIFIC TARGETS

If you have studied any books on nutrition in the past, you have probably become accustomed to seeing lots of numbers (percentage of calories from fat, number of grams of fat) as targets to be sought after in a nutritious diet. While keeping track of your diet in one way or another may be important for certain people at certain times, I don't think that performing any kind of calculation on a daily basis for the rest of your life is the way to go. The important targets are the foods themselves that you will end up including in your lifetime eating plan. In a good plan, the numbers take care of themselves.

I must admit, as the author of *The T-Factor Diet* and co-author of various fat counters, that I have played a large role in focusing attention on the need to reduce fat in the diet for weight management. I suggested that counting fat grams with a specific target in mind was a lot easier than using percentages. It's still true. But I had no intention, then or now, to turn people into human calculators. Counting is a temporary learning strategy. At the start of a new dietary program in which you aim to lower your fat intake, you may need to look up the nutritional values of various foods until you find the ones that appeal to you and which meet your new, lower-fat nutritional objectives. These replace the older, fattier foods. Then you are done with counting and record keeping. The counters remain useful for future reference, when you need information about some new food item.

I have designed the Cancer Prevention Good Health Diet to bring you gradually and naturally, *without counting,* to the nutritional targets that almost all specialists in the prevention and treatment of cancer and heart disease recommend. If you want to *start out* by counting, that's fine. It may give you extra assurance that you are reaching your dietary objectives. You will find a counter in Appendix D, where I will show you how to do the necessary calculations. I have put the nutritional analyses of all recipes in Appendix C. But simply following the one-recipe, one-meal, one-day-at-a-time guidelines will bring you to these objectives within a matter of weeks without the use of a calculator.

Here are the healthful targets for key nutrients:

Fat: Too much fat is the most dangerous nutrient in the American diet. It should be kept to a *maximum* of 20 percent of total calories. The average American diet contains about twice that amount.

Fiber: Too little fiber is associated with elevated cholesterol levels and certain cancers. To achieve the protective effect of different fibers you should consume a *minimum* of 25 grams a day, but 35 grams is better yet. The average American diet includes *less than half the minimal amount.*

Cholesterol: In a generally low-fat diet that is particularly low in animal (largely saturated) fat, dietary cholesterol normally has little impact on blood cholesterol levels. The American Heart Association recommends no more than 300 milligrams a day, a level that should be easily maintained when you follow the Cancer Prevention Good Health Diet.

What about vitamins, minerals, and the important phytochemicals?

When you follow the Cancer Prevention Good Health Diet your consumption of vitamins, minerals, and phytochemicals will equal that found in the diets of people whose risk of cancer is less than half that of the person eating the typical American diet. You will be well in excess of the Recommended Daily Allowances for the key vitamins and minerals that have been found to play a role in the prevention of heart disease and cancer (the best sources for each nutrient are given in Chapter 3). There is no evidence that vitamin and mineral supplementation is required to reach optimum levels.

THE DOS: ACCENTING THE POSITIVE

The most useful guidelines are those that can help you choose the right foods for a nutritious diet. Here is what to aim for:

1. Depending on your total caloric needs, you should eat between 6 and 11 servings of grains (bread, cereals, pasta, rice). Even more if you spend hours at hard labor or other physical exercise. Most of these servings should be of the whole grain, which contains most of the fiber and the entire array of vitamins, minerals, and phytochemicals, much of which is lost in refining.
2. Gradually move toward a total of 9 servings of fruits and vegetables a day. The American Cancer Society recommends a minimum of 5, and that is a good place to start considering that the typical American diet

contains fewer than 2! But 5 servings a day will not provide the protective nutrition to be found in 9 servings.

3. Include at least 3 different colors among the fruits and vegetables each day. Red, yellow/orange, and green are key, but all the colors, from creamy white to magenta, contain valuable phytochemicals. If you eat only one green vegetable on a given day, make it a leafy green, but choose different greens on different days.

4. Include cruciferous vegetables several times a week (broccoli, cauliflower, various cabbages, collards, brussels sprouts, bok choy, mustard greens, kale, kohlrabi, rutabaga, turnips).

5. Include liberal amounts of garlic, onions, leeks, or shallots, either as seasonings for other foods or in greater amounts in combination dishes.

6. Eat at least 1 serving of a citrus fruit each day (but 2 is better).

For many people, these recommendations represent a dramatic change. It's usually best to move slowly toward these goals, since an immediate leap from the typical American diet to this quantity of plant food might make you quite uncomfortable. A diet of this kind contains well over the recommended minimum of 25 grams of fiber each day, but it takes several days, if not 2 to 3 weeks, for your system to adapt. It does this by developing a new and different batch of microorganisms that live in the intestines and deal with the different fibers in a healthful way. I'll have some suggestions on how to deal with bloating in Chapter 7 (page 136).

ARE THERE ANY "BAD" FOODS?

Some dietary experts like to say there are no "good" foods or "bad" foods. It's a question, generally, of quantity. A teaspoon of butter combined with some olive oil can make all the difference in the flavoring of certain dishes that are eaten on special occasions. There's nothing wrong with this. But if the only fat you use is butter, even if you limit yourself to the total fat recommended per day, you are almost certain to be taking in too much potentially harmful saturated fat. The same is true for other foods, such as sugar, red meat, and coffee, which at certain very limited levels may have no dangerous impact. Any more than this should be clearly labeled "bad." Therefore I think it is important to give you some key limitations among my guidelines.

1. Limit the amount of fat you add to food each day. About 1 tablespoon if other fatty foods (cheese, fatty fish, meat) are included in a day's menu, and up to 2 tablespoons if the day's diet is mainly vegetables and

grains. The emphasis should be on monounsaturated fats such as olive, canola, and peanut oils.

2. Limit your consumption of red meat—that is, beef, pork, and lamb. If you are accustomed to daily consumption, begin to omit one day at a time, with an initial goal of cutting intake in half. Then aim for once a week. In my opinion, *optimum intake of red meat is less than once a month or never*. This will become possible once you have discovered enjoyable replacements.

3. Limit fish and poultry to about 6 ounces a day—that's one big main dish, for example, a large fish steak or two pieces of chicken. *You don't need fish or chicken in your diet on a daily basis.*

4. Use primarily low-fat dairy products—for example, 1 percent or skim milk and low-fat frozen desserts. Nutritionists generally recommend 2 servings a day for most adults, to meet calcium requirements, but fish with bones (canned salmon, sardines, jack mackerel) and plenty of whole grains, deep greens, and tofu can substitute for 1 or both of these servings.[2] *(The inclusion of animal protein in the diet increases a person's need for calcium. As you reduce the amount of animal protein in your diet, your need for calcium will also be reduced.)* High-fat dairy products should be used only in small amounts for flavoring special dishes.

5. If you consume soft drinks, including artificially sweetened drinks, begin to replace them with fruit or vegetable juices, water, club soda, or tea, *until they are all eliminated from your diet.* Two or 3 servings of juice or tea each day will make a significant difference in your consumption of beneficial nutrients and phytochemicals.

6. Limit coffee to 2 cups a day; replace coffee with fruit juice or tea. Tea (especially green tea) has such potent protective phytochemicals that some experts suggest counting 2–3 cups of tea as the equivalent of 1 vegetable serving in meeting your vegetable/fruit target for a day.

Now we're ready to get on with the practical, day-by-day implementation of the Cancer Prevention Good Health Diet.

---

[2]Best plant sources of calcium include turnip, beet, dandelion and mustard greens, kale, bok choy, and broccoli. Some brands of tofu are also good sources, but not all. Check the label.

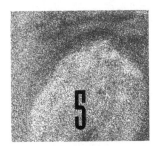

The Cancer Prevention Good Health Diet

PART 2: PRACTICAL IMPLEMENTATION

First Steps

The Cancer Prevention Good Health 3-step plan is meant to remove all pressure and tension from the process of dietary change. Instead of starting with the idea that you have to give up anything, you start by experimenting with different, healthier recipes and methods of preparation. Let things happen as they may by simply keeping the ultimate goal in mind, which is to find delicious combinations of plant foods that taste so good you *prefer* them to some of the less healthful dishes that have been the focus of your present diet.

Here's how you do it.

Think of it as a voyage of discovery. Start by picking out from Chapter 7 two or three recipes that focus on plant foods to try each week over the next few weeks. You want a variety of foods and styles such as pastas and combination dishes that include different vegetables, grains, and legumes. To help you, there is a list of recipes later in this chapter that I think you will find appealing and fun to make during the next several weeks. You don't have to try them in the order listed, or feel limited by my suggestions. Try whatever appeals to you from the recipes in Chapter 7 or pick up any cookbook that emphasizes low-fat plant-food recipes and develop your own plan.

An immediate *daily* goal, which I am sure you can reach without inconvenience or discomfort, *is to include 3 different-colored fruits and/or vegetables.*

These can be side dishes, snacks, or salads as well as main courses. When you do this, you will be over halfway to the minimum objective set by the American Cancer Society (5 servings of fruits and vegetables a day, combined) and a third of the way to the optimum objective of 9 servings a day.

If you are accustomed to eating red meat every day, consider how you might cut that consumption in half. In addition to the plant-food recipes that you will be trying and which might become satisfying substitutes, think in terms of fish or poultry. Chapter 7 contains some delicious fish and poultry recipes (some as simple as throwing a fish steak in the oven to broil), or you might use your own, as long as you keep the fat at a minimum. In a few weeks or months you may find, as my wife, Enid, and I did, that red meat is playing a smaller and smaller part in your diet. About two years ago we realized that we had not had any red meat in the house for several months. We still don't miss it.

Of course, one recipe does not make a meal. Since it might take a couple of weeks of experimentation with new combinations of dishes to make complete satisfying meals on your own, I make a few suggestions for companion dishes along with many of the recipes in Chapter 7. You will also find some suggestions in the meal plans and the "Make a Daily Menu" section later in this chapter.

Do not neglect your leftovers. Fish and poultry from an evening's meal can make good sandwiches or they can be added to a salad the next day. Pasta, combination dishes, and soups are good for lunch—even for breakfast! Don't be bound by tradition or past habits. You can eat anything you like, at any time, in any combination, if it agrees with you. And you can count on your leftovers being nutritious, and part of the Cancer Prevention Good Health Diet.

How to Reach Your Dietary Goals

Your ultimate dietary objectives for plant foods are:

- 9 servings of fruits and vegetables combined
- 6 to 11 servings of grains (bread, cereal, pasta), depending on your caloric needs

These objectives are not as difficult to reach as it might seem. In fact, you'll probably find that they sneak up on you as you cut down on red meat and try new plant-rich recipes. One way to reach them, if you like three main meals and a snack each day, might be:

Breakfast: 2 fruits (juice can count as 1) to go with cereal or toast. But don't forget leftovers or soups. They can count toward your vegetable/fruit as well as your grain targets.

Lunch: 2 vegetables, 1 fruit, and 2 servings of a grain food. If you work away from home and *must* eat out on a daily basis at restaurants where a satisfying variety of these foods is not available, carry your own piece of fruit. If you have refrigeration at your workplace, add some slices or sticks of vegetables.

Dinner: 2 vegetables, 1 fruit, and 2 servings of a grain food.

Snack(s): dried and fresh fruit, grain foods (check out my muffin and other grain recipes).

(These plant-food suggestions assume standard serving sizes and also assume that you will be adding standard servings of fish or poultry several times a week.)

But three square meals is not the only way to go. Many nutrition experts suggest something like a "nibble" plan, which is what I prefer. In the nibble plan you eat a small snack whenever you feel hungry, at any time of the day, and have two small meals and one somewhat larger. For most people the larger meal will fall in the evening, when work, or most of it, is done. To convert the three-square plan to a nibble plan, just transfer some of the plant foods suggested above to snacks between meals. I like fruit most of the time and I always have a large bowl containing a variety of attractive fresh fruit on the kitchen or dining room table. You might prefer a hunk of whole-grain bread, whole-grain crackers, or crunchy vegetables. With three or four snacks of this kind, I think you will find it very easy to hit your daily plant-food goals. And, besides never being hungry, you are likely to remain more alert throughout the day, avoiding both any tendency to feel sleepy after lunch or the late-afternoon blahs.

If you have been eating processed snack foods high in fat and sugar and drinking soft drinks, you will obviously go a long way toward reaching your healthful goal by replacing them with fruits, vegetables, more wholesome grain products, and fruit juices.

Table 5.1 contains a list of foods for which I have been able to find studies demonstrating a preventive impact on cancer either in humans directly, in controlled animal research, or in a test tube (the latter two against experimentally induced lines of cancer cells). This list is expanding almost daily, as more studies appear showing the protective effects of newly investigated phytochemicals. Many of the same foods have a protective impact on heart disease. Just look at all the colors represented in this list! As one nutritionist put it, "Eat a rainbow every day." Build your meals and snacks around the foods on this list; it will light the way to a happier, healthier, and longer life.

Table 5.1 FOODS KNOWN TO CONTAIN PHYTOCHEMICALS THAT MAY PROTECT AGAINST CANCER AND HEART DISEASE

Apple	Licorice root
Artichoke	Mint
Basil	Mustard
Beans, dry	Mustard greens
Bell peppers	Onions
Berries (general)	Oranges
Blueberries	Parsley
Bok choy	Peanuts
Broccoli	Peas
Brussels sprouts	Pineapple
Cabbage	Pumpkin
Cantaloupe	Radishes
Caraway seeds	Red grapefruit
Carrots	Rosemary
Cauliflower	Rutabaga
Celery	Shallots
Chile peppers	Soybeans
Citrus fruits (general)	Soy products
Collards	Spinach
Cucumbers	Squash
Eggplant	Strawberries
Figs	Sweet potatoes
Flaxseed	Tea (green, black)
Garam masala	Tomatoes
(Indian spice mix)	Turnips
Garlic	Walnuts
Grape juice (red)	Watermelon
Horseradish	Whole grains
Kale	Wine (red)[a]
Kohlrabi	Yams
Leeks	

[a]Usually considered separately as an alcoholic beverage, rather than a food. Many experts caution against the inclusion of alcoholic beverages if they are not already a part of your diet, and suggest limiting them to 1 glass of wine for a woman and 2 for a man (per day) in any case.

Specific Mealtime Combinations

THE FOOD PYRAMID

Before going on to some suggestions for meals and menu planning, I think it's a good idea to become acquainted, if you aren't already, with the recent U.S. Department of Agriculture Food Pyramid and to understand what's considered "a serving." When you begin to use combination dishes based on plants as a main course, you will find that these dishes add up to 3 or 4 individual servings of the separate plant ingredients all combined in the one main course. As you examine the pyramid, you may notice that the serving sizes are different from those you are accustomed to. For example, a serving of meat is 2½ to 3 ounces—that's about half the size that many people consider to be a main-course serving, and smaller even than the portions fast-food restaurants put in their larger sandwiches.

I have included the Food Pyramid guide in the box primarily to illustrate recommended numbers of servings and serving sizes in the various food groups, since many people are not aware of these numbers and

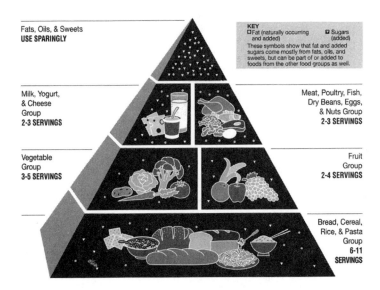

USDA RECOMMENDED NUMBERS AND SERVING SIZES

Bread, Cereal, Pasta, Rice Group

6–11 servings daily; 1 serving = 1 slice of bread, 1 ounce of ready-to-eat cereal, ½ cup of cooked rice or pasta, ½ cup of cooked cereal.

Vegetable Group

3–5 servings daily; 1 serving = ½ cup of chopped raw or cooked vegetables, 1 cup of leafy raw vegetables.

Fruit Group

2–4 servings daily; 1 serving = 1 piece of fruit or melon wedge, ¾ cup of juice, ½ cup of canned fruit, ¼ cup of dried fruit.

Milk, Yogurt, Cheese Group

2–3 servings daily; 1 serving = 1 cup of milk or yogurt, 1½ to 2 ounces of cheese.[a]

Meat, Poultry, Fish, Dry Beans, Eggs, and Nuts Group

2–3 servings daily; 1 serving = 2½ to 3 ounces of cooked lean meat, poultry, or fish; ½ cup of cooked beans, 1 egg, or 2 tablespoons of peanut butter = 1 ounce of meat, or ⅓ serving.[b]

Fats, Oils, and Sweets Group

Use sparingly (fats and sugars occur naturally in foods in the other groups).

Adjust the number of servings according to caloric needs. Generally, older adults and children will be at the lower levels, inactive women below the middle, active women and inactive men around the middle, and teenage boys and active men toward the top.

[a]As I've mentioned before, choosing nonfat or low-fat dairy products will help you to keep the fat in your diet at 20 percent of total calories.
[b]3 ounces of tofu is also equivalent to ⅓ serving.

amounts. However, the recommendations in the Food Pyramid do not take into consideration the specific role phytochemicals other than vitamins and minerals play in the human diet, and the recommendations with respect to total dietary fat and animal foods were not designed to *minimize* the likelihood of cancer and heart disease. They were designed to help the average American meet RDAs for known nutrients in a form most likely to be acceptable to people in our culture. Only about 1 in 10 persons in the United States comes close to consuming the diet recommended in the Food Pyramid.

However, for all the improvement it might bring to the average American's diet, *the Food Pyramid does not go far enough in terms of disease prevention!*

Most experts in the fields of cancer and heart disease prevention feel that the recommendations, which are based on a goal of 30 percent of calories in fat and include too great a focus on animal foods, do not minimize the risk of these degenerative diseases. The preferred goals, which I have stated for the Cancer Prevention Good Health Diet, are only 20 percent of calories from fat with much less emphasis on foods of animal origin.

Now for some specific suggestions.

BREAKFAST

I'm sure you have heard it before: Breakfast is the most important meal of the day. There are mental, emotional, physiological, and nutritional reasons for this statement. People who eat breakfast tend to be more alert and work better throughout the day, avoid late-afternoon letdowns, eat less at night, have better control over their weight, and, on the average, end up with a more nutritious diet than those who skip it.

If you have been skipping breakfast, I suggest that you experiment for about two weeks with my recommendations. It may take that long to become accustomed to making this kind of a change in your eating pattern. When you skip breakfast, your body stops making certain physiological preparations to eat that normally accompany waking. These preparations start an hour or two before you get out of bed. It can take one to two weeks for your system to get charged up again, but making this change may prove to be very important. It will affect your eating pattern over the entire day. You will know in two weeks whether it will work for you for the better. It does for most people. However, if you are one of the rare persons who does not feel better for it, then you should go back to skipping it and plan to add what you might have missed at breakfast at a meal or as a snack later in the day. For example, many people like a bedtime snack of fruit and cereal, which is what some other folks might usually eat for breakfast.

Traditional healthful breakfast suggestions in the United States include a serving or two of a grain food and two fruits—for example, a glass of juice plus some fruit on your cereal. If you happen to be one of those persons for whom citrus fruits do not sit well early in the day, put them off for later, and include another juice (apple, black cherry) or a slice of melon in addition to the fruit you add to cereal. Fruits that go well with cold breakfast cereals include bananas, berries, sliced peaches, and just about any dried fruit—raisins, chopped dates, apricots, prunes. Many of these will work with hot cereal. French toast and pancakes are also excellent low-fat breakfast alternatives, and can be served with fruit or maple syrup. If your cholesterol is over 200 ml/dl, you should limit your egg consumption, if not cut them out entirely.

But don't be limited by tradition! As I mentioned previously, you can eat anything you like, in any combination that agrees with you, at any time of the day. You will be contributing to a nutritious diet when you use any of the leftovers from the main-meal recipes included in the Cancer Prevention Good Health Diet. Many of your leftovers will consist of pasta or other grains, or legumes, in combination with different vegetables. They make excellent, satisfying breakfasts. So do soups. Add a couple of slices of whole-grain bread and a fruit, unless you want to save that for later in the morning.

You might find that whole-grain toast sprinkled with about 1/2 teaspoon of olive oil and a generous amount of garlic and onion powder makes for an interesting combination. For variety, add some crushed marjoram, or other herb. A couple of slices go very well with a cup of coffee or tea. The taste may linger, but it's very satisfying, and, for some reason, using powdered onion or garlic in this way does not leave you with a strong unpleasant breath. Garlic toast made in this way is also an excellent, healthful snack, and it's a good foundation for a sliced-tomato sandwich.

Here are some specific suggestions, from the ordinary to the unusual. They are based on the three-square plan, so, if you prefer to nibble, save a portion of these hearty breakfasts for later in the morning.

GENERIC BREAKFASTS

I

Fruit juice
Cold cereal with fresh or dried fruit
(bananas, berries, sliced peaches, raisins)
Slice of whole-grain bread
Beverage

II

Choice of fresh fruit or juice
French toast or pancakes
(maple syrup or fruit topping)
Beverage

III
Choice of juice or fresh fruit
Hot cereal with dried fruit
Beverage

IV
Choice of fruit
Soup (from an earlier meal)
Slice of whole-grain bread
Beverage

V
Choice of fruit or juice
Serving of a leftover plant-food dish of previous evening
or from freezer
Slice of whole-grain bread
Beverage

Finally, if you'd like to try a supremely nutritious "breakfast in a bowl" look up the recipe for Lee's Power Breakfast (page 94). In addition to being delicious and satisfying, it comes about as close to having everything your body might need to start the day off right as any meal I can imagine.

LUNCH

Where you eat is very likely to influence *the kind* of lunch you eat. At home, with a well-stocked refrigerator and pantry, it's easy to plan for an interesting and healthful variety. If you work outside the home, you may want to consider brown-bagging, using some of the leftovers or homemade soups of your own design. If you can't do this, it's important to have one or more restaurants that you can depend on for serving the foods you like, prepared as you want them, on a daily basis.

Our objective for lunch is to devise several generic menus that you like well enough to make a permanent part of your diet and that include two vegetables and a fruit (on the nibble plan, you save a portion for later). However, you may not want to start adding that much fiber at lunch to a breakfast that has also been fiber rich until your system becomes more accustomed to the changes you are making. If you have been eating a typical American fast-food lunch (a hamburger or ham-and-cheese sandwich with little or no vegetable garnish, french fries, a pastry, and a drink—a lunch which is almost fiber free), you may find it best to make one change at a time.

Even if eating at a fast-food restaurant is most convenient, you are not locked in to a fat-laden, fiberless meal. Many fast-food restaurants are responding to the public's interest in healthful eating and are providing one or two lower-fat sandwiches and a basic salad topped with different kinds of meat, cheese, or cold seafood. But the choice will always be limited compared with sit-down restaurants that offer many different vegetables, salads, and luncheon-size entrees of pasta, fish, and poultry. If you eat at the same fast-food restaurant every day, you may end up always having to order the same things, and that can be terribly boring. Since healthful dessert offerings also are usually very limited, you can improve matters greatly by carrying fruit with you for dessert (as well as for snacks). If you must eat at a fast-food restaurant every day, locate more than one, so that you can find a more healthful and satisfying variety of foods.

Here are some generic luncheon recommendations that are meant to serve as guidelines. You will soon have some delicious and nutritious leftovers from your dinners, which, if you brown-bag it, can replace the main items in these generic suggestions. Your leftovers will tend to be much more interesting than the generic suggestions and will make packing a lunch well worth the effort. The attractive colors and appetizing aromas of your brown-bag lunches will generate a lot of interest among your colleagues.

Be flexible—if you aren't able to have 2 different vegetables and a fruit with lunch, or you wish to follow the nibble plan, include whatever you omit as a snack, or at a meal later in the day. For example, at dinner, instead of a large (6-ounce) serving of fish or poultry, have a smaller (3-ounce) portion and a double or triple serving of a plant food.

GENERIC LUNCHES

I

Fruit or vegetable juice
Sandwich of your choice
Vegetable side dishes or garnishes
Fruit dessert
Beverage

II

Soup
Sandwich with vegetable garnishes
or
Luncheon salad

Fruit dessert
Beverage

III
Large luncheon (vegetable) salad
Whole-grain bread or roll
Fruit dessert
Beverage

IV
Fruit or vegetable juice
Luncheon-size portion of fish or poultry
Small dinner salad or side of cooked vegetable
Beverage

V
Large luncheon pasta/vegetable salad
Roll or whole-grain bread
Fruit
Beverage

DINNER

For most people in the United States the evening meal is the main meal, and, except perhaps for weekends, it's when most people do their home cooking. This is the time to experiment with different dishes. Here are the steps you should follow at dinnertime to put the Cancer Prevention Good Health Diet into practice.

Step 1. Try at least two new main-course recipes each week. As your main courses, choose from the following list of combination dishes that use fish or chicken together with grains, vegetables, or legumes, or which consist entirely of plant foods, such as the meatless pastas, legumes, and grains. (Check them out in Chapter 7 before you begin, to see which ones appeal to you most. Some serve equally well as side dishes, in smaller portions of course.)

Tuna Casserole *(page 130)*
Onion Quiche *(page 132)*
Stuffed Winter Squash *(page 133)*
Escarole Torte *(page 130)*
Southwest Casserole *(page 131)*
Tamale Pie *(page 133)*

Monna's White Chili (*page 134*)
. Mock Lasagna (*page 145*)
Once-a-Week Pasta (*page 150*)
Spinach Lasagna (*page 148*)
Dave's Rich and Zesty Burritos (*page 137*)
Dave's Rich and Zesty Tostados (*page 138*)
Barley and Vegetables (*page 142*)
Couscous, Chickpeas, and Vegetables (*page 139*)
Black-Eyed Peas and Greens (*page 140*)
Spiced Tofu Loaf (*page 156*)
Scalloped Potatoes and Tofu (*page 153*)
Curried Tofu and Cabbage (*page 154*)
Potato-Tofu Casserole (*page 154*)
Broccoli Walnut Stir-Fry (*page 155*)

I want in particular to encourage you to try the tofu recipes. As a person who was never fond of tofu until my wife put in the effort to find tasty ways to prepare it, I can assure you these are delicious and loaded with those special protective phytochemicals that are more abundant in soybeans than in any other food.

Some of the above recipes contain a variety of different plant foods and can serve either as complete meals or as main courses with one or two side dishes. When combining dishes, you will do well to add a non-starch vegetable side dish or a salad to a starchy main course, or a starchy side dish (such as a grain or potato) to a non-starch main course. You can start or finish your dinner with a serving of fruit. You'll find some suggestions to help you complete your dinner menu with many of the recipes in Chapter 7.

Step 2. On other days, when you are using a fish or poultry main course and not trying a new recipe, include 2 vegetables, either as side dishes, in a salad, or in combination. Here are some general guidelines for the quick and easy preparation of vegetable side dishes or salads:

(a) Just about any vegetable, from asparagus to zucchini, can be steamed or microwaved (or simmered if necessary in a small amount of boiling water). Some vegetables, like beets and winter squash, can simply be baked. Before serving, add just a smidge of oil—for example, olive oil—plus your preferred herbs or spices. A single teaspoon of oil is often enough for a bowl containing 4 servings. It provides just enough fat to bring out the flavor of your herbs and spices and it gives vegetables the texture that makes them enjoyable.

(b) When you prepare a small dinner salad, use at least three different-colored vegetables and add a bit of your favorite salad dressing if one of my own recipes is not handy. (A ½ cup of chopped vegetables or 1 cup of leafy vegetables is considered a serving.)

(c) Use a low-fat method of preparing your fish or poultry main course. If you don't have a preferred method, my basic fish and poultry recipes in Chapter 7 take only about two minutes to prepare. It's hard even to call them "recipes," since these basic methods use only a few herbs and spices, and sometimes a little oil.

What about dessert?

Fruit is generally your best choice for dessert, but I'm also a great fan of frozen yogurt and like to nibble on popcorn after dinner, in place of a dessert. Frozen yogurt is a good source of calcium, and, if you like it and don't include other dairy products in your diet, a daily serving of a low-fat frozen yogurt would not be out of line. But I also want to show you that eating in a healthful way does not mean giving up "sweets." In the dessert section of Chapter 7 you will find some mouthwatering recipes for a few cakes, pies, and brownies which demonstrate that healthful desserts can taste good, too.

GENERIC DINNERS

Now for the outlines of some complete dinner menus.

There are three general approaches. One focuses on plant foods that are normally used as a main course. These are often starchy dishes, with either cheese or an animal food in combination with plant foods. For example, in the meals where you try one of the 20 recipes in the list above, a complete generic dinner might look as follows:

I

Fruit appetizer
Cancer Prevention Good Health main course
(Spinach Lasagna, or another recipe from the list above)
Side vegetable or salad
Serving(s)[1] of whole-grain bread
Choice of dessert
(Fruit, if not included as an appetizer, or frozen yogurt,
or your choice from the recipes in Chapter 7)

---

[1]Your grain servings, from 6 to 11 per day, should be adjusted to your caloric needs.

This would, of course, be a much larger meal than you would include in the nibble plan. Dessert and appetizer might be included there as snacks.

A second approach uses a fish or poultry main dish (or meat on rare occasions), with 2 vegetables and a fruit. For example:

II

Fish, poultry, or (rarely) meat course
2 vegetable side dishes
or
1 vegetable and a small dinner salad
Serving(s) of whole-grain bread
Choice of fruit dessert

Of course, rather than prepare your main and side dishes separately, you can toss your fish, poultry, or meat in a pot with a selection of vegetables and make a stew, similar to what I suggest among my recipes.

A third variation of a generic dinner will occur more and more frequently as you become accustomed to a plant-based diet. As you learn to prepare plant-based meals, cooking vegetables and grains in tasty ways will become easier and take much less time. You will know the recipes of the ones you like best "by heart," and you will want to make quantities that can suffice for more than one meal. Once cooked, they can be stored in the refrigerator for 2 or 3 days, and can be frozen for longer periods. Having these available will make it more convenient to design meals that contain 3 or even more plant-food dishes. You will have to prepare only one or at most two fresh recipes at any given time, to which you will add a favorite leftover or two. And the leftovers, especially combination dishes, improve with a day or two of age. I think you will be surprised at how the transition to this way of eating occurs, if you follow my suggestions, *and don't try to accomplish it too quickly.* Just keep going at it, one recipe, one meal, one day at a time.

With this many plant foods in your main meal, you may not want to add fruit for an appetizer or a dessert. It certainly won't be needed to meet preventive goals. If you desire something sweet for dessert, I suggest frozen yogurt or one of my own low-fat dessert recipes in Chapter 7.

III

3 or more plant-based dishes
Whole-grain bread or roll
(optional, depending on nature

of plant-based dishes)
Choice of dessert

Make a Daily Menu

Making a daily menu with the Cancer Prevention Good Health Diet is simply a matter of mixing and matching your preferred meals and snacks to reach the goals for plant foods. In the three-meal-plus-snack plan, you can start by choosing and combining from among the various generic mealtime menus in the preceding pages. As I suggested previously, you might aim for 2 fruits for breakfast, 2 vegetables and 1 fruit at both lunch and dinner, with plant-food snacks to round it out or to make up for omissions at one or another meal. You also include 2 or more grain servings with each meal, or fit them in as snacks. Your ultimate objective is to reach 9 servings of vegetables and fruits each day, and between 6 and 11 servings of grain foods (depending on caloric needs). You may include even more plant foods on days when you do not include fish, poultry, or meat.

It may be even easier to meet plant-food goals on the nibble plan, especially after you have been following the Cancer Prevention Good Health Diet for a few weeks. By that time you will almost always have a leftover or two that can contribute to prevention goals. You will have no problem reaching Cancer Prevention Good Health goals for plant foods after you have replaced overly processed fat-laden snacks with fruit, and as your emphasis in main meals switches away from meat to vegetables, legumes, and grains. A serving of nuts or seeds, while listed in the meat (or protein) group in the Food Pyramid, can also serve as a healthful snack, as well as an ingredient in combination main dishes. Nuts and seeds are loaded with protective antioxidant phytochemicals, but because of their high fat content, 1 serving (that is, 1 ounce) a day is enough.

Should You Keep a Record When You Begin the Cancer Prevention Good Health Diet?

Record keeping is not an essential part of the Cancer Prevention Good Health Diet. If you follow the recipes and meal plans I've just suggested, you will soon be eating a nutritious diet without counting anything. The idea is to make plant foods the central focus of your diet according to the guidelines I've just laid down.

However, if you would like to monitor your progress for a while, until your new diet becomes second nature, you might find it useful to keep a record. If weight loss is not your highest priority, all you have to keep is a rough eating diary. At the end of each day, write down what you have eaten and continue to do so until you are satisfied that you are following Cancer Prevention Good Health guidelines. You can use the form in Figure 5.1 (and photocopy it, if you like). I will suggest a more detailed record in the next chapter if quick weight loss is your goal.

Figure 5.1 EATING DIARY

Write down what you have eaten today, being sure to indicate size of serving (see Food Pyramid on pages 53–54). Then total the number of fruits and vegetables (aim for 9 servings, but you may begin with 5) and grains (aim for between 6 and 11, according to your caloric needs). Then circle the colors (y = yes, n = no) to make sure you are consuming the variety recommended. Pay attention to the additional guidelines in the lower right-hand corner of the record.

Breakfast_____   Total number vegetables   _____
          _____   Total number fruits   _____
          _____   Total number grains   _____
          _____

Lunch   _____   Color of fruits and vegetables:
          _____   Red   y   n   Yellow/ y   n
          _____   Orange
          _____   Green   y   n   Other   y   n

Dinner   _____   Additional guidelines:
          _____   2 servings of low-fat dairy products or other
          _____   sources of calcium; limit of 6 ounces of fish
          _____   or poultry; limit of 1 tablespoon of added
          _____   fat.

Snacks   _____
          _____
          _____
          _____
          _____

Must You Approach the Goal Gradually or, If You Prefer, Can You Make Changes Quickly?

As I will explain in the next chapter, if quick weight loss is your immediate goal, yes, you will need to make changes quickly. And even if weight loss is not your highest priority, you can move as quickly as suits your personal style. One of my concerns is that a sudden increase in your intake of fiber might make you temporarily uncomfortable. However, if you are willing to endure some discomfort, your system will adjust, although it may take as long as a week or two.

Some people, usually a small minority, find it easier to make drastic rather than gradual changes in their diets. For them, making a drastic change illustrates commitment.

But there are dangers ahead. The likelihood of failure is great because there are so many things to be done, all at once. Drastic changes are easier to do in a "boot camp" setting, under supervision, or where there is overwhelming support from a like-minded group. On your own, where many different foods and new methods of preparation are entailed, where there may be little social support (if not outright resistance) and the major burden of change is on your shoulders, the cards can be stacked against you.

With that said, if you wish to implement the Cancer Prevention Good Health Diet as quickly as you can, here is some advice.

1. Read the whole book and have a clear grasp of the entire program of diet and exercise, and of any other recommendation that has relevance for you (for example, dealing with stress), before you begin.
2. Lay out your week's menu, and your shopping list.
3. Be sure to include in your planning everyone on whom your dietary changes (and possible activity changes) will have some impact. If you prepare food for several family members, you may create an explosive situation if, overnight, you introduce an entirely new cuisine. And if you rely on someone else to prepare your meals, and your needs are different from others in the family, your requests may be greeted with irritation and resentment. Deal with these possibilities in advance.

Some Final Words

Whether you use my preferred gradual approach, or the more drastic one I've just discussed, the changes you are about to make are not likely to be done in complete isolation from other people and other activities. Understanding from family and friends can be critical—they need to be aware of what you intend to do and why. While it's usually possible to sneak in two or three new dishes every week without fanfare, just as you might any other new recipes, I think you will get more support from other family members, especially children, if you include them in meal planning, making shopping lists, and the actual cooking.

Then there is the question of eating out. Whether you move ahead gradually or quickly, you will want to make sure you can order meals that are consistent with the Cancer Prevention Good Health Diet when dining out. This may mean finding new restaurants and engaging your servers in some discussion about the menu. Most sit-down restaurants are able and pleased to modify a number of different dishes on their menus in exactly the way you'd like them.

SUGGESTIONS FOR ETHNIC DINING

Here are some suggestions for what to select as **best bets** (√) and what to **avoid** ⊘ to make choices consistent with prevention guidelines within various ethnic cuisines.

CHINESE

√ Chicken in foil as an appetizer.

√ Steamed dumplings (Peking raviolis).

√ Authentic Chinese restaurants make most menu items to order so you can ask questions about method of preparation and use of fats, and which vegetables are contained in each dish.

√ Steamed vegetables, chicken, tofu, lean meats, and seafood dishes in light broth-based or wine sauces.

√ Stir-fried (specify as little oil as possible) vegetables, chicken, tofu, lean meats, and seafood dishes. Examples: moo goo gai pan chicken, shrimp with snow-pea pods, boned chicken or lobster cantonese, moo shu chicken, shrimp, or vegetables.

√ Ask if it's possible to substitute shrimp, scallops, or chicken in place of pork or beef in menu entrees.

√ Wonton soup or other clear, broth-based soups.

√ For dessert, fresh pineapple, orange sections, or fruit bowl with fortune cookie.

⊘ Fried items such as batter-dipped appetizers, spareribs, fried rice, "crispy" beef, egg foo yung, and chow mein noodles.

FRENCH

√ Consommé or other broth-based soup as appetizer.

√ Steamed, poached, roasted, or grilled fish or chicken—for example, coq au vin (chicken in wine), pot-au-feu (stewed chicken), bouillabaisse (fish stew), or poached quenelles (steamed fish dumplings).

√ Dishes served "en papillote" (steamed in a paper envelope).

√ Steamed or sautéed (in wine, broth, or tomato sauce) vegetables served à la carte rather than vegetables served with hollandaise, butter, or cream sauce. Ratatouille is a lower-fat vegetable dish.

√ Sherbet, fresh fruit, or pears in wine sauce for dessert.

⊘ Fatty sauces such as hollandaise, béarnaise, béchamel, beurre blanc, velouté, and Mornay; "au gratin" or "en casserole" items; items in a pastry shell; croissants; quiche.

INDIAN/PAKISTANI

√ Mulligatawny or lentil (Dahl rasam) soup.

√ Chapati (unleavened bread) and nan (leavened bread) are preferable bread choices as many Indian bread items are fried.

√ Items prepared without frying or added ghee (clarified butter).

√ A curry dish made with chicken, lobster, shrimp, lentils, or vegetables.

√ Combination vegetable plates (several offered on a large tray, with condiments).

√ Order plain rice or use a rice dish as a main entree.

√ Mango or papaya slices or Indian fruit cocktail as dessert.

⊘ Fried breads, coconut soup, and coconut cream.

I T A L I A N

√ Pastas served with tomato-based sauces that do not contain meat. Marinara, pizzaida, and pomodoro sauces are good choices. Clam or calamari sauces are also a tasty, lower-fat alternative to meat or cream sauces.

√ Baked or broiled chicken (without skin), veal cutlet, or fish dishes topped with meatless tomato-based sauces and minimal or no cheese. For example, chicken piccata or cacciatore.

√ Seafood sautéed in wine rather than oil—for example, scampi al vino blanco (shrimp sautéed in white wine sauce).

√ Minestrone, consommé with pastina, or cioppino (seafood soup) as an appetizer or for lunch.

√ Fresh Italian bread without butter, rather than garlic bread.

√ Italian ice.

⊘ Antipasto salad, Italian sausage, Alfredo and other cream sauces, cheesecake, and dishes made with lots of high-fat cheese, meat, or oil (meat lasagna, manicotti, parmigiana, cannelloni, pesto).

P I Z Z A

√ Vegetable toppings, not meats. Traditional pizza toppings such as pepperoni and sausage are loaded with saturated fat. The meat actually cooks atop the pizza with all the grease being absorbed into the sauce and crust. If the opportunity arises, just take a look at the cardboard that has held pizzas with different toppings—you'll see a big difference in the amount of grease in the bottom of pizza boxes that held a meat pizza versus a vegetable one.

√ Ask for extra sauce and half the ordinary amount of cheese.

⊘ High-fat meats (pepperoni, sausage, ground beef) and extra cheese.

√ Clear soups, like miso soup, as an appetizer.

√ Sushi and sashimi.

√ Hibachi chicken.

√ Steamed, grilled, or broiled chicken, or fish teriyaki style.

√ Ask if shrimp, scallops, or chicken can be substituted for pork or beef in menu entrees.

√ Mandarin orange sections, sherbet, and fresh fruit are low-fat dessert selections.

⊘ Fried bean curd, tempura, other foods battered and fried, agemono, and katsu dishes.

M E X I C A N

√ Salsa, salsa verde, picante sauce, or taco sauce as a topping or dip rather than guacamole or sour cream.

√ Black bean soup or gazpacho as an appetizer or for lunch. Hold the sour cream.

√ Tortillas or soft tacos (unfried) filled with chicken, seafood, or vegetables. Refried beans in a restaurant are generally loaded with lard, but not always, so ask. Good choices include chicken or seafood burritos, or enchiladas, if you can get them with half the usual amount of cheese.

√ Side orders of soft flour tortillas, black beans (these are usually low in fat, in contrast with refried beans), or Mexican rice.

√ Seafood or chicken in tomato-based or vegetable sauces—for example, camarones de hacha (shrimp in tomato coriander sauce) or arroz con pollo (boneless chicken breast with rice).

√ Order à la carte low-fat items and vegetables—combination dinners are usually served with refried beans, sour cream, guacamole, cheese, and fried foods.

√ Many Mexican restaurants have begun offering a variety of spicy salads, but they are not always on the menu, so ask if they will make a salad to order.

√ Fresh pineapple or baked bananas for dessert.

⊘ Sour cream, guacamole, fried items like chimichangas, tostadas, and tortilla chips, and items with lots of cheese or fatty meats.

MIDDLE EASTERN/GREEK

√ Skim-milk yogurt and cucumber soup.

√ As an entree, choose grilled or baked items like shish kebab (more restaurants are offering kebabs with chunks of fish steaks rather than red meat), baked fish with tomatoes and rice, or oven-braised chicken with kumquats.

√ Pita bread.

√ Fruit compote or poached apples for dessert rather than baklava, kataif, or rice pudding.

⊘ Pastries and items rich in cheese or eggs.

TIPS FOR AIRLINE TRAVEL

If you are about to take a flight and a real meal rather than a snack will be served, you will usually find that the airline will offer a variety of choices to suit the needs of different travelers. In addition to kosher, low-sodium, and low-cholesterol meals, they almost always serve fruit plates at any meal, including breakfast, and cold seafood plates for lunch or dinner. These fit right in with the Cancer Prevention Good Health Diet, and, in my experience, compared with the hot meals, they are always clearly superior.

For breakfast, most airlines are already offering cereal, low-fat milk, and fruit in place of eggs and sausage. But if that breakfast is not available, pancakes will have less fat than the egg dish, and they'll taste better, too.

When you make reservations, or at least 24 hours before takeoff, call the airline to see if a meal will be offered and what special plates will be available on your flight. I do a great deal of traveling and never order anything other than the fruit plate (with cottage cheese) or the cold fish plate for lunch or dinner. If you cannot obtain a meal to your liking, carry your own brown bag. I see more and more people doing this now that the airlines have cut back on meals in flight. If a meal is not to be served, it's a good idea to take something decent along for a snack. While you will usually get an apple with an airline snack (often rosy red in color, but green in taste), the meat sandwich and packet of processed cheese certainly don't make the grade.

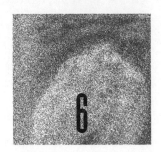

The Cancer Prevention Good Health Express: Weight Loss in a Hurry (for Those Who Need It)

If you are more than 20 percent overweight according to the chart in Table 6.1, I can sympathize with you in your desire to lose weight. People who are more than 20 percent over recommended weight for their height carry around with them a significantly increased risk for both heart disease and certain cancers, as well as for virtually all other degenerative diseases. The most recent study shows that risk of heart disease for American women in their middle years may actually begin to increase with every pound over a weight that is *15 to 20 percent **below** the weight of the average woman.* The same is true for cataracts, and most likely heart disease, for men. Evidently, using the charts in Table 6.1 as a reference, health risks increase with every pound over the very lowest figure in each range. And these charts, based on the Metropolitan Life Insurance Tables, recommend weights that are many pounds *below* the unfortunately inflated suggested weights in the 1990 U.S. Department of Agriculture/Department of Health and Human Services table, which I also include for your reference in Table 6.2.[1]

In addition to the health risk, most overweight people don't like the way

---

[1]While being thin may help you reach the age of 70, once you get there, a recent study reports that being too thin is more dangerous than being as much as 20 pounds over normal weight. The suggested-weight tables are designed to predict mortality for persons in their younger and middle years, and not the elderly. Having a few extra pounds of fat after the age of 70 may give a person the extra energy needed to fight off the illnesses that occur with increasing frequency after that age.

Table 6.1 SUGGESTED WEIGHTS FOR ADULTS, METROPOLITAN LIFE INSURANCE COMPANY (1959)[a]

HEIGHT Feet	Inches	Small Frame	Medium Frame	Large Frame
Men				
5	2	128–134	131–141	138–150
5	3	130–136	133–143	140–153
5	4	132–138	135–145	142–156
5	5	134–140	137–148	144–160
5	6	136–142	139–151	146–164
5	7	138–145	142–154	149–168
5	8	140–148	145–157	152–172
5	9	142–151	148–160	155–176
5	10	144–154	151–163	158–180
5	11	146–157	154–166	161–184
6	0	149–160	157–170	164–188
6	1	152–164	160–174	168–192
6	2	155–168	164–178	172–197
6	3	158–172	167–182	176–202
6	4	162–176	171–187	181–207
Women				
4	10	102–111	109–121	113–131
4	11	103–113	111–123	120–134
5	0	104–115	113–126	122–137
5	1	106–118	115–129	125–140
5	2	108–121	118–132	128–143
5	3	111–124	121–135	131–147
5	4	114–127	124–138	134–151
5	5	117–130	127–141	137–155
5	6	120–133	130–144	140–159
5	7	123–136	133–147	143–163
5	8	126–139	136–150	146–167
5	9	129–142	139–153	149–170
5	10	132–145	142–156	152–173
5	11	135–148	145–159	155–176
6	0	138–151	148–162	158–179

[a]The weights in these tables are based on lowest predicted mortality for persons at ages 25–59. The weights were calculated for fully dressed persons, and include 5 pounds for men and 3 for women; in both cases, heights were calculated including 1-inch heels.

The Cancer Prevention Good Health Express: Weight Loss in a Hurry

Table 6.2 SUGGESTED WEIGHTS FOR ADULTS, UNITED STATES DEPARTMENT OF AGRICULTURE AND UNITED STATES DEPARTMENT OF HEALTH AND HUMAN SERVICES (1990)[a]

| Height[b] | Weight (pounds)[c] | | | |
| | 19 to 34 years | | 35 years and over | |
	Midpoint	Range	Midpoint	Range
5'0"	112	97–128	123	108–138
5'1"	116	101–132	127	111–143
5'2"	120	104–137	131	115–148
5'3"	124	107–141	135	119–152
5'4"	128	111–146	140	122–157
5'5"	132	114–150	144	126–162
5'6"	136	118–155	148	130–167
5'7"	140	121–160	153	134–172
5'8"	144	125–164	158	138–178
5'9"	149	129–169	162	142–183
5'10"	153	132–174	167	146–188
5'11"	157	136–179	172	151–194
6'0"	162	140–184	177	155–199
6'1"	166	144–189	182	159–205
6'2"	171	148–195	187	164–210
6'3"	176	152–200	192	168–216
6'4"	180	156–205	197	173–222
6'5"	185	160–211	202	177–228
6'6"	190	164–216	208	182–234

[a]The higher weights in the ranges generally apply to men, while the lower weights more often to women. The difference results from the larger muscle and bone mass in men at each height. The higher weights for persons 35 and older reflect the opinion that as people age they might be able to carry more weight without endangering their health. Recent research questions this assumption, except possibly for people 70 and over, for whom a few extra pounds can supply energy to put up a stronger fight against the illnesses that occur with aging.
[b]Without shoes.
[c]Without clothes.

they look (I didn't when I was 60 pounds overweight some 30 years ago) and they find it a lot harder to move around carrying more than a few extra pounds of fat (I couldn't climb a flight of stairs without becoming short of breath). When you add to this list the discrimination many overweight people experience in the workplace and in social situations, the conclusion is inescapable: thin is in. In fact, thinner than thin seems even better.

So, yes, it may be a good idea to lose some weight, and I can understand your desire to do it as quickly as possible. Since losing quickly always requires at least a little inconvenience if not some sacrifice, I can also appreciate your need to see some noticeable progress in order to remain motivated. There's nothing quite like the feeling you get when you begin to swim around in clothes that were formerly pretty tight!

What Is Your Best Weight?

But before you go rushing off to fulfill some scientist's statistical projections, which are meant to apply to the population as a whole and not to any one individual, you need to ask yourself, "What would my own, personal, healthiest weight really be?"

I can answer that for just about everyone, and most likely for you without even knowing or seeing you. It has little or nothing to do with your bathroom scale.

Your best weight is the weight you will ultimately reach when you eat the low-fat, plant-rich diet that I'm recommending in the Cancer Prevention Good Health Diet and get physically active on a daily basis, burning the number of calories the human body was designed to burn through millions of years of evolution, before the advent of labor-saving (but life-threatening) devices.[2]

Only some compelling, unusual health problem makes for an exception to this prescription for an individual's personal-best, healthiest weight.[3] If you must achieve a lower weight for professional reasons—for

[2]Health officials and scientists have devised other measurements for relating body build and composition to a person's health and the likelihood of disease. The body-mass index, or BMI, is computed by the formula "weight in kilograms [kg] over height in meters squared [m²]." An index greater than 27.8 for men and 27.3 for women is indicative of obesity. The waist-to-hip ratio is another measurement that correlates with heart disease, stroke, and diabetes. To find your waist-to-hip ratio, measure your waist near your navel while standing in a relaxed posture, without pulling in your stomach. Measure your hips over your buttocks at the largest point. Divide the waist measurement by the hip measurement. A ratio of 0.80 or less is recommended for women, and 0.95 or less for men. The larger your belly in relation to your hips, the greater the risk. You may also see recommendations for percentage body fat. While the recommendations for men seem reasonable and reachable (14–18 percent), those for women are not. The usual recommendation for women (18–22 percent) does not take into consideration the true sex differences in body-fat requirements between males and females, related to the child-bearing process, which tend to result in about 10 percent more body fat per weight in women compared with men. Male or female, your best body-fat percentage is that which you will reach when you eat a nutritious diet and engage in physical activity on a daily basis.
[3]There is a rare form of hyperlipidemia in which the system cannot handle carbohydrate properly. Having lived long enough to be reading this book, you should already know if this applies to you and be under a doctor's care. Other reasons for modifying the advice that is appropriate for the average, healthy adult would be in the treatment of an already existing disease, such as after a heart attack or in the effort to contain certain cancers.

example, if you are a professional long-distance runner, ballerina, or fashion model—and your target weight requires extreme caloric restriction and hours of intense exercise on a daily basis, you may only be injuring your health in the long run.

So, if your goal is to reach your personal-best weight quickly rather than in the gradual way that would occur over time as you adopt the Cancer Prevention Good Health Diet and build an active lifestyle, how can you do it in a manner that assures both good health and permanency?

The Weight-Loss Express

You should not kid yourself into thinking you can go on a special, very-low-calorie diet, losing several pounds a week, and then, when you reach your goal, hop off that diet onto a "maintenance plan" that has little or nothing to do with the way you lost your weight in the first place. If you've done this before, you should know that this only leads to wide swings in your weight which, by analogy, seem to defy the laws of gravity—you end up higher rather than lower a short time down the road.

For permanent weight management, the way you lose weight must be harmonious with the way you intend to keep it off. As you lose your weight you must find, and enjoy, the foods and methods of preparation that you will live with thereafter to maintain your losses. If you are a sedentary person, physical activity must become as essential to your daily activities as brushing your teeth. If that seems highly unlikely to you at the present moment, I think I can show you (Chapter 9) how to become active in a way that fits your temperament, work schedule, and social obligations. You will feel so good about being active that you will become just as uneasy missing a day of activity as you do when you fail to brush your teeth!

HOW TO USE THE CANCER PREVENTION GOOD HEALTH DIET TO LOSE WEIGHT QUICKLY

To lose weight quickly in a way that's consistent with principles that lead to the prevention of degenerative diseases, and to do it in a manner that leaves you with a permanent weight-management program *already in place* when you reach your goal, *you should do everything I have suggested in previous chapters for implementing the Cancer Prevention Good Health Diet.* The only differences are:

1. You make some of the changes in your diet more quickly.
2. You set an explicit, average, daily target for total calories and a fat-gram goal that will equal 20 percent of that total.

3. You keep track of calories and fat grams to ensure a more dependable rate of weight loss.

In a moment I'll give you instructions about how to do this, but first I want to answer a question that is usually foremost in a person's mind who wants to lose weight quickly:

HOW FAST CAN I EXPECT TO LOSE?

You will lose several pounds the first week. That would occur with any diet that has several hundred fewer calories per day than your present diet. While it's primarily water weight (overweight people tend to store several extra pounds of water compared with lean folks), it will feel good since you will be able to stick a few fingers under your belt if it's been a bit snug. Thereafter, you can expect to lose about 1 to 2 pounds a week if you are about 20 percent overweight. You will lose somewhat faster during the first few weeks if you are more than 30 percent overweight.

You should not lose weight more quickly than the rate I am recommending; if you do, you may make it almost impossible to maintain your losses.

If you lose weight too quickly you may suffer a serious decrease in your metabolic rate. It can be so serious that after several weeks or months of weight loss you require 10 to 20 percent fewer calories at your new, lower weight than the average person for whom that identical weight has been their normal weight. This reduction in caloric need may persist for an indefinite period of time, perhaps months or years. In addition, after too quick a weight loss, certain fat-incorporating enzymes may become hyperactive, incorporating fat into your fat cells much more voraciously than normal. It's no wonder that people who lose weight too quickly almost always end up fatter than ever within a year or two.

Any decrease in metabolic rate is also prevented through physical activity. By combining the Cancer Prevention Good Health Diet with daily activity you may actually be able to increase your metabolic rate (see Chapter 9). To reach your best, healthiest weight, and, more important, to maintain that weight, requires physical activity of some kind *every day,* unless you begin to engage in some very vigorous sport or become temporarily ill. Then days off are appropriate.

3 SIMPLE STEPS TO LOSE WEIGHT QUICKLY

Cutting fat to 20 percent of calories and beginning to eat a plant-rich diet almost always means eating fewer calories and much more bulk, that is, much more food in total volume. For example, a ½ cup of greens or other leafy vegetable contains fewer calories than a pat of butter. All by itself, cutting fat and increasing plant foods usually results in eating a couple of hundred calories a day less than previously and in a gradual weight loss that averages one-half to two-thirds of a pound a week for most people who are 20 percent overweight or more.

Losing weight more quickly requires that you upset your daily energy balance a little more dramatically. Since a pound of stored fat contains about 3500 calories, to average 1 to 2 pounds a week in weight loss over a period of weeks or months, you must withdraw from your fat storage an average of between 500 and 1000 calories a day. In general, women can achieve this by cutting calories to 1200 a day, while men should cut to 1800 a day.

To do this in a way that results in full implementation of the Cancer Prevention Good Health Diet as well as permanent weight loss, you do the following:

1. Begin immediately to follow my suggestions in Chapter 5 for basic breakfasts and lunches, saving one of the fruits, vegetables, or grains for a snack to use when you feel hungry between meals.
2. Time permitting, begin experimenting with three or more new recipes each week from my list on pages 59–60, to speed the full implementation of the Cancer Prevention Good Health Diet. You may lose 10 to 20 pounds in the next 2 to 3 months and you must have your new way of eating in place to maintain that loss.
3. In addition, you must keep track of fat grams and calories. The targets for losing weight are, in round figures:

	UPPER LIMITS	
Women	30 grams of fat	1200 calories
Men	40 grams of fat	1800 calories

Follow the instructions in Appendix D, and use the counter and the handy eating diary that are printed there, to help you meet these goals. You must write everything down for *at least 3 weeks*. If you are unsure of serving sizes, weigh and measure everything until you know what standard measures really look like. While just about everyone underestimates total calorie intake by approximately 20 percent, recent research shows that overweight people are especially likely to underestimate ("forget") their fat intake.[4] That's just one of the reasons I suggest you pay special

---

[4]In a study done several years ago by my colleagues at Vanderbilt University, even trained dietitians underestimated their fat intake by as much as 20 grams a day, which is equal to 180 calories in fat.

attention to fat grams and write things down. Once you are *sure* you know the fat and calorie contents of the foods, and the new low-fat methods of preparation that are becoming permanent parts of your diet, you can stop. But only then.

Although you can use a tablespoon of added fat, and sometimes more, as spread and in cooking when you are not making a special effort to lose weight, at the reduced calorie levels that it takes to lose quickly you may need to eliminate almost all added fat.

Warning: do not go below 20 grams of fat daily. Your body needs a certain minimum amount of fat for essential metabolic functions. First signs that you have cut too low include chapped lips, rough skin, or brittle hair.

If you are acquainted with my earlier work on weight management, *The T-Factor Diet,* you may notice that I am recommending somewhat lower levels of fat as the upper limit in the Cancer Prevention Good Health Diet. That's because I want you to become accustomed to keeping fat at 20 percent of total calories, not only while losing weight but thereafter. My purpose is to help you cut your risk of cancer and heart disease in every way possible in addition to losing weight. When you reach your weight goal, 20 percent of calories will be more like 40 grams a day for most women (assuming a diet of about 1800 calories), and 50 grams for most men (assuming a diet of about 2250 calories). Once you have incorporated the foods and methods of preparation in the Cancer Prevention Good Health Diet in your own diet I hope you will not find it necessary to continue to count anything.

HOW TO ASSURE YOUR SUCCESS

Here are a few hints to help assure your success.

Never Go Hungry. While I suggest a diet of 1200 calories a day for women and 1800 for men, it is not necessary for you to feel hungry to succeed. You should always be able to have something to eat when you are hungry. Although most people find that the increased volume of plant foods more than compensates for the decrease in fat calories, some people do get hungry every few hours on a low-fat diet. If that applies to you, it's not at all unhealthy. Just follow my nibble plan. Choose nutritious plant foods (fruits and vegetables) to nibble on so that in case you exceed your daily target it will not be by very much.

Here is a suggestion based on my personal experience.

When I made up my mind to lose weight back in 1963, I decided that I needed at least one fallback food that I could eat at any time, day or night, if I felt the urge. I chose grapefruit, and I would peel and eat one whenever I felt hungry (or most of one—they are very filling). I still use a similar, although somewhat modified and relaxed, strategy. To this day I keep a bowl of fruit in plain sight, filled with whatever looked good at my last visit to the supermarket. Today's bowl contains apples, oranges, grapefruits, bananas, and grapes (I finished the plums yesterday).

Just about any fruit or non-starchy vegetable will do for nibbling. They are mostly water (as much as 90 percent or more) and loaded with healthful fiber. Other concentrated carbohydrate foods, such as breads and cereals (especially the latter with added dried fruit and nuts), are not as good. Because they are "dry foods," they contain more calories per unit of weight than fresh fruits and vegetables. In addition, the cereals usually contain some fat and are scientifically sweetened to a point where the factory's testers indicated they were most tasty. In other words, they are designed to turn on your appetite, not necessarily satisfy it.

Get Family and Friends on Board. When people fail in changing their eating habits it's often because family and friends fail to understand what they need to do to be helpful, and fail to cooperate. You should explain what you are about to do, and why, to all persons on whom a change in your lifestyle will have an impact. The suggestions I made on pages 65–66 will help you obtain the cooperation you need to be successful.

Learn to Deal with Negative Emotions without Turning to the Wrong Foods. If you turn to eating under stress of any kind, it's most likely that you turn to something loaded with fat or sugar, or both. While you attempt to find other ways to deal with stressful situations, the most immediate thing you need to do is *find some nonfat, non-sugar foods to turn to.* Then, if my suggestions for dealing with stress in Chapter 9 don't help, you may want to resolve, once and for all, the problems that lead you to fail in managing your weight by getting some professional help. In the meantime, *there is no need to kick yourself for chomping on fatty, sweetened foods when you are stressed out.* There are biochemical reasons why these foods (especially chocolate-flavored ones) seem to temporarily assuage negative emotions; they affect calming, pleasure-sensing parts of the brain. For your health's sake, however, you must find other ways to do this that don't result in obesity!

WHY YOU CANNOT EAT ALL YOU WANT OF FAT-FREE FOODS AND MAINTAIN YOUR WEIGHT LOSS

Here I must give you some extra words of warning: You cannot eat all you want of foods just because they contain little or no fat and continue to lose weight. In fact, it is possible to gain weight on any food if you continually outeat your energy needs day after day. It's just a lot harder to do this on carbohydrate or protein than on fat, but not impossible. The reason is that dietary fat requires little work to transform it into the form your body needs for storage. If you overeat on fat, about 97 percent of the calories will end up in your fat cells. Carbohydrate and protein need a lot of work to transform them into the form of fat that can be stored, so that only 75 percent of their calorie content gets into your fat cells. This gives you a little insurance when you are eating a plant-rich diet. The insurance is even greater if any extra carbohydrates come from fruits and vegetables because of the fiber: high-fiber foods go through your system faster and fewer of the calories are absorbed. Many people double their number of bowel movements when they increase fiber from the American average of about 11 grams a day to the 25 or more that will occur with the Cancer Prevention Good Health Diet. Instead of lingering for as long as 48 hours in the system, food begins to pass through in 24 hours, or less (an action that also results in a lowered risk of colon and rectal cancer).

Beware of processed "no-fat" foods.

I'm thinking particularly of so-called fat-free cookies and other highly sweetened snack foods, desserts, and pastries. These foods often contain a list of artificial ingredients that, if laid end to end, would reach from your chin to your navel. Many of them are added to mimic the feel and taste of fat in the mouth, and a few of them may actually contain fatty acids, such as lecithin, monoglycerides, and diglycerides. These fatty acids don't have to be included on the label as contributing to the fat content. These "fat-free" foods also may attempt to make up for the attractiveness of fat by containing more sugar, corn syrup, or high-fructose corn syrup than a fatty version. Because some people who adopt a low-fat diet think they can eat anything that contains no fat and not gain weight, they begin to eat several portions of no-fat products instead of a single portion of a fat-containing version.

Let me give you an example of what the end result of thinking and acting this way might be.

A serving of one popular brand of coffee cake contains 5 grams of fat and 250 calories, while another, fat-free version contains less than 0.5 gram of fat per serving and 190 calories. Let's say, for the sake of argument, that you could eat a piece of that fat-free coffee cake containing 190 calories at dinner tonight and not gain weight. But you choose two pieces because they are "fat-free." This means that you take in a total of 380 calories, which, of course, is a surplus of 190 calories. Because, as I explained earlier, the body does work harder to convert carbohydrate to fat than it does to convert dietary fat to body fat, only about 143 of these surplus calories (75 percent) get converted to fat for storage. However, you could have had a piece of the "real thing," with 5 grams of fat and only 250 calories. That's just 60 surplus calories and even if all of them got stored as fat, you'd be better off.

What is even worse, however, is that the label on the fat-free version may not always be accurate. In one case, where I had a "fat-free" coffee cake tested in the laboratory, it contained 1.5 grams of fat per serving size indicated on the label, which is considerably over the legal limit for a fat-free cake. In addition, everyone without exception to whom I showed this cake and asked what they would serve themselves as a single serving indicated that they would cut a piece about double the size of the little sliver suggested by the food processor. Voilà: 3 grams of fat and 380 calories. A few people said that once they got started they would probably eat half the cake, which in this case would have been equal to 4 servings. I should point out, in defense of the manufacturer, that variations in fat content can happen unintentionally when a new shipment of the grains used in the product contains more fat than the original shipment used in testing the recipe for labeling purposes. Oats, wheat, and other grains can vary slightly according to variety or as a result of different growing or milling conditions.

Setting a Weight-Loss Goal and Maintaining Your Losses

If you are 20 percent or more over your goal weight I believe you will be most successful if you set an intermediate target for weight loss. I believe that target should be just 10 percent of your present body weight no matter how overweight you are. There are several reasons for this:

1. A weight loss of just 10 percent of your body weight can make a significant difference in your cholesterol level and blood pressure, and it can result in a significant reduction in your risk of heart disease, stroke, cancer, and diabetes.
2. It is important to learn what it takes to maintain your losses. Practicing maintenance periodically as you proceed in steps toward your ultimate goal will make it easier in the end to maintain all of your losses.
3. You will learn at which weight you feel most comfortable, physically and psychologically. That's the weight you should maintain, without regard for your scale and any weight table.

4. You should not attempt to reach any weight that you can't live with comfortably because constant efforts to restrain yourself lead to frustration and failure. And while there is some debate over just how physiologically dangerous repeated cycles of losing and gaining weight can be, there is little question that failure to maintain a weight loss is damaging from a psychological and emotional perspective.

Of course, my goal has been to show you how to lose weight in a way that helps guarantee maintenance. Stick to the guidelines I have outlined in this chapter and start using the recipes that follow. In a few weeks I believe you will find the Cancer Prevention Good Health Diet as easy to follow as your present diet, but best of all, you will like it as much as or more than your present diet. That's your guarantee of maintenance.

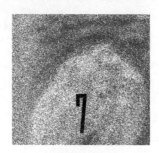

Recipes

Before You Start

Before you start to experiment with some of these new recipes, I'd like to give you some hints that may make improving your diet easier and more enjoyable.

I think it's important that you do everything you can to make preparing food just as pleasurable as eating it. Many times, when I'm preparing something especially attractive to the eye as well as to the palate, I feel like a da Vinci in the kitchen. If I am not producing a "masterpiece," it's at least a working sketch. Every day is a new creation, even when I'm preparing dishes I've made many times before. The foods are new, fresh, and colorful, and the urge invariably hits me to vary my seasonings or to add another ingredient that happens to catch my eye.

To really enjoy preparing food, I think you should bear in mind that although certain dishes take more care than others, recipes are not mathematical formulas. For me, recipes are just convenient guidelines that open the door to my own creativity. I hope you will enter into this spirit of cooking, if you haven't already. Some of my favorite dishes, such as Cauliflower du Barry, are based on recipes a couple of hundred years old or more, which required a certain inventiveness. These recipes simply advised the user to blend certain ingredients. Often, only very rough guidelines for quantity were given. Old-time cooks evidently would take the basics and add seasonings and possibly other ingredients according to availability or to suit their tastes. And, of course, without the availability of refrigeration, shopping for fresh ingredients and then cooking them were normally affairs that took considerable time.

Cooking in the old-time way today, especially for people who work away from home, is pretty difficult. Coming home close to dinnertime and starting a meal from scratch, when you're tired or have family members calling in to the kitchen every few minutes demanding to know when dinner will be ready, doesn't lend itself to the calm, enjoyable preparation of new recipes. Here are some hints that might make cooking an easier, more pleasurable task.

First, some basics. You must have the right equipment.

Treat yourself to good utensils.

Knives. You need sharp knives that keep their edge and make it possible for you to cut, chop, and mince with the least possible effort. A minimum would include (with approximate measurements, since blades may vary a bit among manufacturers):

10-inch slicing knife (a thin blade for slicing turkey, for example)

8- or 10-inch chef's knife (for the chopping jobs, or splitting a winter squash)

6½-inch utility knife (sometimes better on the larger vegetables such as carrots, potatoes, and cabbages than a paring knife or chef's knife)

4-inch paring knife (I like two because they are in constant use)

My favorite knives are made by Henckels or Wüsthof and they are a pleasure to use.

Keep your knives in a wooden knife block conveniently near the place on your counter or chopping block where you work, and, by all means, *keep them sharp.* More accidents occur with dull knives than with sharp ones because of the difference in effort involved. And it's no fun to have to fight with your food to prepare it. I like ceramic sharpening sticks, or stones. Give your knives a few swipes on the stick each time, just before you use them, and every so often you should go through the process of putting a new edge on them. If you don't know how, and there were no instructions with your stick, ask at your cutlery store.

Pots, Pans, and Casseroles. Big combination dishes, pasta, and casseroles often require large utensils. I suggest, as a minimum:

2- and 3-quart saucepans (with covers)

6-quart covered stockpot (can be used for pasta as well as stews, soups, and chilis)

6-, 10-, and 12-inch skillets

3½- and 5-quart casseroles (oven and microwave safe)

Also handy are a small assortment of baking dishes and muffin tins and a roasting pan large enough for chicken and turkey. By all means have a baking pan suitable for lasagna (approximately 8 × 11 × 2 inches for serving 6, but, if you like lasagna and begin to serve more and more plant-based recipes, it's worth having a special lasagna pan for parties, about 10 × 14 × 4 inches, so that you can serve 12).

I prefer a skillet to a wok on my electric stove top for stir-frying, but the product is not quite as crispy and flavorful as you will get when you use a wok (my stove warns against using a wok on the electric element). You may be able to find a skillet-wok specially designed for use on an electric stove at your cutlery store.

Miscellaneous. It's a good idea to have an assortment of serving spoons, spatulas (the kind that will not scratch your pots and pans), and other implements handy near the stove. I keep mine upright in a canister, looking like a bouquet, right next to the stove. A blender and a food processor are indispensable—I think you need both, as well as a big wooden salad bowl (for example, about 4 inches deep and 14 inches across the top for everyday use, larger for company). And, finally, a cutting board that's easy to keep clean, a pepper mill, and, if not a special spice grinder, at least a mortar and pestle for grinding herbs, spices, and seeds (for example, Garam Masala, page 181, and all-purpose Herb Salt, page 183).

Plan your meals ahead of time as much as possible, and be organized in your kitchen and in your cooking technique. A few more hints:

1. Obviously, if you are about to prepare new recipes, you must decide which ones for any given day and you may have to shop for ingredients—plant foods are usually best fresh. You may need a new assortment of herbs and spices. So, a shopping list is called for.

   You may have to find a convenient day with a little extra time to cook new recipes since it may take a little longer to put unfamiliar things together. And new recipes usually require some thought about accompanying dishes (suggestions in a moment).
2. It's much more pleasant to cook in a well-organized kitchen. Just in case

you haven't given this much thought, make sure the pots, pans, and casseroles that you are going to use most frequently are in convenient places. You may be pulling out utensils you haven't used much in the past now that you are preparing more plant-based recipes.

3. Keep your preparation space as uncluttered as possible and organize your utensils and your ingredients before you start to cook. This ranks right up with the most important advice I can give you for making cooking a pleasant experience. If you don't already do it for recipes requiring more than a few ingredients and one pot, try this just once: Before you begin, lay out (on your uncluttered counter and stove tops) each mixing dish and pot that you will need for the recipe. Then lay out each ingredient that you will use in the recipe in the order called for. If you have been accustomed to playing hide-and-seek with your ingredients and utensils in the middle of preparation, making an assembly line of this kind is going to make a tremendous difference in your tension level!

Let me give you a quick example: I suggest you try my Spinach Lasagna (page 148) early in your conversion to a plant-based diet. You will need your lasagna pan and another large pan to soak your lasagna noodles. You will be coating each layer of noodles with sauce, followed by fresh spinach, basil, mushrooms, and three kinds of cheese. If you have everything arranged in a semicircle around your lasagna pan, you go zipping around (I go left to right) with no fuss, no mess, and no confusion.

Making Interesting Menus with Plant-Based Recipes

When you first begin your gradual introduction to the Cancer Prevention Good Health Diet you can, for many of your meals, use the traditional "meat and three" idea. These menus are conceptually easy to design. When people think of meat they usually think of red meat. Now, of course, many people are eating more poultry and fish. And the "three" should be two cooked vegetables and a starch, or a small salad, cooked vegetable, and a starch. You can always use this traditional model for many of your menus, using mostly fish and poultry, rather than red meat. Remember to vary your vegetables, using different colors and including the important cabbage and *Allium* (onion and garlic) families. In the vegetable and salad sections of this chapter, I'll give you some quick and simple suggestions for preparing your side dishes whenever you plan a meal of this kind.

But our goal is to move more and more toward complete plant-based menus, and to menus that use animal foods only as complements or garnishes to primarily plant-based dishes.

BALANCING A PLANT-BASED MENU

Here the principle is also simple: When the main dish is primarily starchy foods (that is, largely grains, legumes, or pasta) and is not a complete meal in itself, you look for non-starchy side dishes. When the main dish comprises non-starchy plant foods, you include a starchy side dish. Naturally, if the meal is entirely or mostly plant based, you will be consuming several servings of the size stipulated in the USDA Food Pyramid. As more meals of this kind begin to form the focus of your diet, you will soon reach or exceed the goal of 9 standard servings of vegetables and fruits daily. As you may recall from the Food Guide on page 53, standard servings of cooked non-leafy fresh vegetables as well as legumes are ½ cup, while leafy fresh vegetables are 1 cup. A plant-based meal will have as many as 4 or 5 such servings all by itself.

Some examples will make this clear.

Among the list of main dishes on pages 59–60 that I suggested you try are some that contain a large proportion of starchy plant foods or legumes, and others that do not. Among the starchy main dishes, some are fully satisfying as meals in themselves and provide a variety of different plant foods, while others serve best accompanied with some side dishes. A few contain poultry or fish as a garnish. Here is a list of these, with some generic suggestions that can apply to similar dishes of your own concoction. Your appetite should determine whether you add everything I suggest, and take into consideration the foods you have eaten (or plan to eat) at other times of the day.

The primarily starchy main dishes include:

Tuna Casserole	Southwest Casserole
Stuffed Winter Squash	Tamale Pie
Monna's White Chili	Mock Lasagna
Once-a-Week Pasta	Spinach Lasagna
Dave's Rich and Zesty Burritos	Barley and Vegetables
Dave's Rich and Zesty Tostados	Couscous, Chickpeas, and
Black-Eyed Peas and Greens	Vegetables
Potato-Tofu Casserole	Scalloped Potatoes and Tofu

With these you would add non-starchy cooked vegetables and/or a salad. Leafy greens and cruciferous vegetables are at the top of the list, but you will find recipes for carrots, celery, eggplant, beets, and others in the vegetable section of this chapter.

Primarily non-starchy main dishes include:

Onion Quiche	Meatless Meat Loaf
Escarole Torte	Spiced Tofu Loaf
Curried Tofu and Cabbage	Broccoli Walnut Stir-Fry

With these you add one starchy side dish, along with any other cooked vegetable or salad, according once again to your appetite and the foods you have eaten at other times of the day.

In addition to these starter recipes, you will find others just as appealing, so be sure to check out the entire chapter.

Concise Guide to Herbs and Spices

The judicious use of herbs and spices can add a great deal to your cooking and eating pleasure. I keep the ones I use most frequently in a wine-style rack at the rear of my work area, and others on revolving shelves in the cabinet above, one shelf for seeds, another for liquids, and a third for infrequently used items. I have compiled this guide from various sources, often from different recipes that looked particularly interesting (although I haven't gotten around to trying them all).

I suggest you try each seasoning either one at a time or in simple, limited combinations, to see what you like best. All foods can be seasoned in a variety of ways, each quite distinctive. For example, I have found recipes suggesting that carrots fare well with the addition of bay leaves, caraway seed, celery seed, chervil, chives, curry powder, dill seed, dill weed, ginger, mace, marjoram, nutmeg, savory, tarragon, and thyme, in addition to pepper and parsley. So, while using pepper and parsley, I might add just one of the others when preparing carrots as a side dish. (For completeness, I have included references to meats in this guide even though I hope to discourage you from including meat to any great extent in your diet.)

Allspice—meats, fish, gravies, relishes, tomato sauce

Anise—fruit

Basil—green beans, onions, peas, potatoes, summer squash, tomatoes, lamb, beef, shellfish, eggs, sauces

Bay Leaf—artichokes, beets, carrots, onions, white potatoes, tomatoes, meats, fish, soups and stews, sauces and gravies

Caraway Seed—asparagus, beets, cabbage, carrots, cauliflower, coleslaw, onions, potatoes, sauerkraut, turnips, beef, pork, noodles, cheese dishes

Cardamon—melon, sweet potatoes

Cayenne Pepper—sauces, curries

Celery Seed—cabbage, carrots, cauliflower, corn, lima beans, potatoes, tomatoes, turnips, salad dressings, beef, fish dishes, sauces, soups, stews, cheese

Chervil—carrots, peas, salads, summer squash, tomatoes, salad dressings, poultry, fish, eggs

Chili Powder—corn, eggplant, onions, beef, pork, chili, stews, shellfish, sauces, egg dishes

Chives—carrots, corn, sauces, salads, soups

Cinnamom—stewed fruits, apple or pineapple dishes, sweet potatoes, winter squash, toast

Cloves—baked beans, sweet potatoes, winter squash, pork and ham roasts

Cumin—cabbage, rice, sauerkraut, chili, ground-beef dishes, cottage or cheddar cheese

Curry Powder—carrots, cauliflower, green beans, onions, tomatoes, pork and lamb, shellfish, fish, poultry, sauces for eggs and meats

Dill Seed—cabbage, carrots, cauliflower, peas, potatoes, spinach, tomato dishes, turnips, salads, lamb, cheese

Dill Weed—vegetables, salads, poultry, soups

Ginger—applesauce, melon, baked beans, carrots, onions, sweet potatoes, poultry, summer and winter squash, beef, veal, ham, lamb, teriyaki sauce

Mace—carrots, potatoes, spinach, summer squash, beef, veal, fruits, sauces

Marjoram—asparagus, carrots, eggplant, greens, green beans, lima beans, peas, spinach, summer squash, lamb, pork, poultry, fish, stews, sauces

Mustard—asparagus, broccoli, brussels sprouts, cabbage, cauliflower, green beans, onions, peas, potatoes, summer squash, meats, poultry

Mustard Seed—salads, curries, pickles, ham, corned beef, relishes

Nutmeg—beets, brussels sprouts, carrots, cabbage, cauliflower, greens, green beans, onions, spinach, sweet potatoes, winter squash, sauces

Oregano—baked beans, broccoli, cabbage, cauliflower, green beans, lima beans, onions, peas, potatoes, spinach, tomatoes, turnips, beef, pork, veal, poultry, fish, pizza, chili, Italian sauces, stews

Paprika—salad dressings, shellfish, fish, gravies, eggs

Parsley Flakes—all vegetables (especially potatoes), soups, sauces, salads, stews, eggs

Pepper—most vegetables, meats, salads

Poppy Seed—salads, noodles

Rosemary—mushrooms, peas, potatoes, spinach, tomatoes, vegetable salads, beef, lamb, pork, veal, poultry, stews, cheese, eggs

Saffron—rice

Sage—eggplant, onions, peas, tomato dishes, salads, pork, veal, poultry, ham, cheese

Savory—baked beans, beets, cabbage, carrots, cauliflower, lima beans, potatoes, rice, squash, egg dishes, roasts, ground-meat dishes

Sesame Seed—asparagus, green beans, potatoes, tomatoes, spinach

Tarragon—asparagus, beets, cabbage, carrots, cauliflower, mushrooms, tomatoes, salads, macaroni-and-vegetable combinations, beef, poultry, pork

Thyme—artichokes, beets, carrots, eggplant, green beans, mushrooms, peas, tomatoes, pork, veal, poultry, cheese dishes, fish, stuffing

Turmeric—mustards and curries, chicken

Breakfast Foods

There are a number of healthful breakfasts in addition to that good old standby: hot or cold cereal, fruit, toast, and coffee or tea. Many people don't realize that pancakes and French toast can be excellent low-fat alternatives. I have found that Egg Beaters works just as well as whole eggs in recipes for these two breakfast foods, and several of my favorite recipes follow. Lee's Power Breakfast is an especially hearty way to start the day. I go for simplicity, however, and I am fond of a plain hunk of whole-grain bread and coffee, reserving my fruit for later in the morning. I sometimes use a bit of olive oil on a thick piece of toast, sprinkled with garlic and onion powder. As I mentioned elsewhere, it goes fine with sliced tomato, and can be seasoned with one of a number of herbs (rosemary, basil, thyme, and oregano are my favorites).

But don't neglect leftovers. If it's available, appeals to you, and agrees with you, start the day with a bowl of soup or any leftover plant-based dish that happens to be in your refrigerator. A bowl of warm pasta may feel much more satisfying if you've been accustomed to eggs, bacon, and fries and wish to improve your diet by increasing the number of plant foods.

Basic Pancake Mix

ᴥ

For a homemade, nutritious pancake mix that's hard to beat for flavor and texture, you can mix together the dry ingredients listed below and store the result in an airtight container. There will be enough for 8 full recipes of 12 pancakes each. Add the Egg Beaters, milk, and oil when you're ready to cook a batch.

THE MIX

4 cups whole-wheat flour
3 cups all-purpose flour
1½ cups low-fat soy flour
2 cups wheat germ

1 teaspoon salt
1 cup instant nonfat dry milk
⅓ cup baking powder

THE PANCAKES

1½ cups mix
½ cup Egg Beaters
1 cup skim or 1% milk or water

1 tablespoon oil
Nonstick vegetable cooking
 spray (optional)

1. Combine the mix with the Egg Beaters, milk or water, and oil. The batter is best left slightly lumpy.
2. Heat a Teflon pan, or other pan sprayed with cooking spray, over medium heat. Pour about ¼ cup of batter per pancake into the pan.

When the cakes are bubbly on top and brown on the bottom, flip them and brown the other side. ✌

Makes 12 pancakes, 6 servings.

Brancakes

¼ cup Egg Beaters
2 cups skim or 1% milk
¾ cup All-Bran or Bran Buds
   cereal

1½ cups all-purpose flour
1 tablespoon baking powder
¼ teaspoon salt
2 tablespoons sugar

1. Mix the Egg Beaters together with the milk and then stir in the cereal. Let stand 5 minutes.
2. Stir together the flour, baking powder, salt, and sugar in a medium mixing bowl. Add the cereal mixture, stirring to combine, and let stand 5 minutes.
3. Drop the batter, using ¼ cup for each pancake, onto a lightly greased, preheated griddle. Cook, turning once, until golden brown on both sides. ✌

Makes 12 pancakes, 6 servings.

French Toast

This is good served with fresh fruit, applesauce, or a sprinkle of powdered sugar to go with the cinnamon. Of course, it's hard to beat a tablespoon or two of real maple syrup, but it doesn't need any butter.

¼ cup Egg Beaters
2 tablespoons skim or 1% milk
¼ teaspoon cinnamon

2 slices whole-grain bread
Nonstick vegetable cooking
   spray

1. Mix together the Egg Beaters, milk, and cinnamon. Dip the bread in the mixture, coating both sides.
2. Spray a skillet with nonstick cooking spray, and heat over medium heat. Fry the bread in the pan, turning once, until golden brown on both sides. ✌

1 serving.

Corncakes

↦

1⅓ cups yellow cornmeal
⅓ cup whole-wheat flour
⅓ cup all-purpose flour
2 teaspoons sugar
2 teaspoons baking powder
Dash of salt

¼ cup Egg Beaters
1 cup skim or 1% milk
1 tablespoon vegetable oil
1 teaspoon honey
Nonstick vegetable cooking
  spray

1. Combine the dry ingredients in a medium-sized bowl.
2. In another bowl, mix together the Egg Beaters, milk, oil, and honey.
3. Spray a griddle or skillet with cooking spray, and heat over medium heat. When hot, spoon batter into pan to make pancakes about 4 inches in diameter. Cook until they begin to bubble and are golden brown on the bottom. Turn them over and cook until done. ↦

Makes 8 corncakes, 4 servings.

Lee's Power Breakfast

(for Two)

↦

Here is a rich, hearty breakfast of fruits, cereals, grains, seeds, and yogurt all mixed in a single bowl. It's a phytochemical feast! Dr. Lee Fleshood makes it about twice a week when he expects a late lunch and says it keeps him happy and free of hunger longer than any other breakfast.

2 cups water
6 ounces either frozen blackberries, blueberries, or cherries
⅓ cup each raisins, raw sunflower seeds, and pumpkin seeds
1 cup old-fashioned oatmeal
Mueslix or whole-grain cereal
Honey or maple syrup (optional)
Plain or vanilla nonfat yogurt
Choice of sliced banana, peach, strawberries, or apple (optional)

1. Put the water, frozen fruit, raisins, and seeds in a 2-quart saucepan and bring to a boil.
2. Add the oatmeal and cook for 5 minutes.

3. Thicken to preferred consistency with Mueslix or other cereal.
4. Divide into 2 servings and, if desired, add honey or maple syrup to sweeten.
5. Cover with a layer of yogurt.
6. Add a layer of sliced banana, peach, strawberries, or apple (optional). ✦

2 servings.

Soups

I like soup just about any time of the day. Sometimes I have a cup of leftover soup for breakfast, and I often have a cup at other times of the day as a snack. Don't be afraid to try some of the recipes below at what might, at first, seem unusual times to have a cup of soup. You may become a convert. And, if you are trying to manage your weight, you may find that you'll eat less and have an easier time of it if you have a cup of soup before your main meals. Be sure to check out my Soup of the Day recipe—it's just as good as my Once-a-Week Pasta (page 150), and another great way to empty your refrigerator crisper.

Soup of the Day
✦

This is a potpourri of whatever you can find in the crisper. It can be fresh, new vegetables, but you can also use anything that looks just a bit beyond the point that you'd want to use it in a salad. I've used virtually every kind of just-over-the-hill vegetable at one time or another. I usually add something starchy to my broth or bouillon base to give it body—for example, barley, rice, or lentils if I'm making only a small amount of soup, or a potato, chopped in small pieces, in a larger recipe. You may find it worthwhile to make enough for several full-cup servings. If I don't have any homemade broth, I use Wyler's bouillon powder or cubes, at half strength. (The primary ingredient in regular bouillon is salt; it can contain from 800 to 1500 milligrams of sodium per cube or teaspoonful.)

FOR A SMALL AMOUNT OF SOUP START WITH
1 cup chicken broth (or bouillon)
2 to 3 tablespoons rice, barley, or lentils

AND ADD

Whatever appeals to your fancy from the refrigerator—greens,
onions, carrots, cabbage, broccoli, and so on—but don't add more
than your liquid will cover
Sprinkle of thyme, marjoram, or other of your favorite herbs
Salt to taste (if not using a regular bouillon cube)
Fresh-ground black pepper to taste

Bring to a boil, reduce heat, and simmer on low until vegetables are done.
For larger amounts, you can double or triple the broth base and add a
potato chopped in small pieces and whatever else strikes your fancy. ❧

*Serving size is 1 cup; your total recipe will tend to vary
considerably depending on choice and amounts of ingredients.*

Celery Soup
❧

1 whole bunch celery, sliced thin, including leaves	6 cups bouillon or stock
	1 teaspoon dried basil
1 onion, sliced thin	¼ teaspoon ground black pepper
3 cloves garlic, minced	Salt to taste
1 fresh tomato, cubed	1 tablespoon lemon juice
1 tablespoon olive oil	

1. In a large saucepan, partially covered, braise celery, onion, garlic, and
   tomato until onion is wilted and translucent.
2. Add all other ingredients and bring to a boil.
3. Lower heat and simmer until celery is tender, about 1 hour. ❧

8 servings.

Clam Chowder
❧

Cornstarch will add a little body to soups made with low-fat milk. The
milk we use in our soups is a locally produced ½% variety that's fortified
with milk solids and has a fuller flavor and texture than regular skim milk.
Try it if it's available in your supermarket.

2 cans minced clams, drained,
reserving juice
Enough water to add to clam
juice to make 2 cups
1 medium potato, cut in ½-inch
chunks
2 stalks of celery, sliced thin
1 onion, chopped

1 clove garlic, minced
1 cup 1% milk
3 tablespoons cornstarch
½ teaspoon salt
¼ teaspoon thyme
½ teaspoon paprika
Ground pepper to taste

1. Cook the potatoes, celery, onion, and garlic with clam-juice-and-water mixture until tender.
2. Combine the milk and cornstarch and blend well.
3. Add the clams, seasonings, and milk/cornstarch to the cooked vegetables.
4. Simmer, stirring, until the mixture thickens to your preferred consistency. ✺

6 servings.

Curried Squash/Cauliflower Soup
✺

This is one of our unusual soups. It may seem like a strange concoction, but give it a try. It's been a great success with our tasters and at our dinner parties. Freezing will not harm the flavor, and when we make it for ourselves we store half in the freezer for future occasions.

2 tablespoons olive oil
1 head cauliflower, coarsely
chopped
1 large onion, chopped
4 cups chicken bouillon, divided
2 cups cooked butternut or
acorn squash, pureed
1 teaspoon salt

2 teaspoons turmeric
1 teaspoon coriander
1 teaspoon chili powder
1 teaspoon ginger
1 teaspoon thyme
½ teaspoon cumin
Ground black pepper to taste

1. Put the oil in a 6-quart pot. Add the cauliflower and braise over low heat, partly covered, for about 5 minutes.
2. With a slotted spoon, lift the cauliflower into a bowl and set aside.
3. Add the onion to the pot and braise until translucent.
4. Add 2 cups of the bouillon and simmer, covered, for 15 minutes.

5. Lift the onion out with a slotted spoon and puree in a food processor or blender.
6. Return the onion to the broth.
7. Add the remaining bouillon and the cauliflower, squash, and spices.
8. Simmer, covered, for about 30 minutes or until the cauliflower is tender.
9. Correct the seasonings and serve. ⊕

6 servings.

Cold Cucumber Soup
⊕

As with other cold soups, this one is very refreshing on a hot summer's day.

3 cucumbers, peeled and seeded
1 tablespoon butter
1 leek, sliced, discarding tough upper leaves (although these may be saved for other soups, stews, and pasta sauces)
1 bay leaf
1 tablespoon flour

3 cups chicken bouillon
1 teaspoon salt
1 cup 1% milk
1 teaspoon dried dill
Juice of ½ lemon (1 tablespoon)
Pepper to taste
½ cup low-fat sour cream

1. Shred or grate 1 of the cucumbers. Set aside and chill.
2. Melt butter in a 3-quart saucepan. Cube the remaining cucumbers and sauté them in the butter with the leek and bay leaf over medium heat for 2 or 3 minutes.
3. Reduce heat to medium low, partially cover, and continue cooking for 20 minutes, stirring occasionally.
4. Stir in the flour.
5. Add the bouillon and salt. Cover and simmer for 30 minutes.
6. With a slotted spoon, lift the vegetables out and puree them in a blender or food processor.
7. Return them to the stock and add the shredded or grated cucumber and the milk, dill, lemon juice, and pepper to taste.
8. Chill well and serve with a dollop of sour cream. ⊕

6 servings.

Chilled Tomato-Orange Soup with Avocado

A gazpacho-style soup made even more interesting than most by the addition of citrus fruit.

2 shallots, chopped
2 cloves garlic, minced
2 fresh green chiles, seeded and diced
¾ inch of fresh ginger, peeled and minced
1 tablespoon olive oil
2 pounds fresh tomatoes, quartered
Juice of 1 orange
Juice of 1 lime
½ teaspoon dried basil
½ teaspoon salt
Ground pepper to taste
1 medium avocado, peeled, pitted, and diced

1. Put the first 4 ingredients in a food processor and process until smooth.
2. Put the oil in a small skillet, heat, and add the shallot/garlic/chile/ginger mixture. Cook over low heat, stirring now and then, for about 4 minutes.
3. In the meantime, put the tomatoes in the food processor and puree them.
4. After 4 minutes or so, add 1 cup of the pureed tomatoes to the skillet. Bring to a boil; then reduce the heat and let the mixture simmer for about 6 minutes.
5. Put the remainder of the tomatoes and the fruit juices, basil, salt, and pepper in a bowl.
6. Add the skillet mix to this and blend.
7. Add the diced avocado and mix.
8. Chill until very cold. ✺

6 servings.

Chicken, Chard, and Rice Soup

~

We've become very fond of Swiss chard, but you can use just about any kind of leafy cabbage or other greens in this recipe.

About 1½ pounds Swiss chard
   (approximately 2 bunches)
1 tablespoon butter
1 tablespoon oil
1 medium onion, chopped
6–7 cups chicken broth

¾ cup brown rice
½ cup grated Parmesan
1 tablespoon minced parsley
Salt and pepper to taste
Extra Parmesan for garnish
   (optional)

1. Wash the chard well and cut coarsely into strips (include stems).
2. In a large pot, melt the butter, add the oil and onion, and sauté over medium heat until tender.
3. Add the chard and stir to coat. Cover the pot and heat about 4 minutes to wilt it.
4. Add the broth and bring to a boil.
5. Add the rice, cover, lower heat, and simmer until the rice is done (about 45 minutes). Stir occasionally and add more broth as necessary.
6. When the rice is done, add the Parmesan, parsley, salt, and pepper.
7. Serve sprinkled with more cheese, if desired. *~*

6 servings.

Mushroom Soup

~

While we like to cut our mushrooms to size, you can do it much more easily in a food processor. You can also take out a portion of the soup and puree it in a blender just before you add the cornstarch, return it to the soup, and continue. This step gives the soup an even richer texture and is worth the bother.

1 tablespoon butter
2 bunches scallions, chopped
2 cloves garlic, crushed
4 cups chicken broth
1 pound mushrooms (medium
   size), cut in half and sliced ¼
   inch thick

Salt and pepper to taste
4 tablespoons cornstarch
2 cups milk
¼ cup chopped fresh parsley

1. In a 3-quart saucepan sauté the scallions and garlic in the butter until translucent.
2. Add the chicken broth and bring to a boil.
3. Add the mushrooms, salt, and pepper. Lower the heat and cook about 15–20 minutes.
4. Meanwhile, dilute cornstarch in a small amount of water and blend well.
5. When the mushrooms are done add the cornstarch, stirring constantly.
6. When the mixture begins to thicken, add the milk and parsley, stirring constantly until heated. *Do not boil.*
7. Correct the seasonings and serve. ✤

8 servings.

Beet and Cabbage Borscht
✤

Although my parents liked borscht and prepared different versions from recipes brought over with them from Europe, there was something about the color and the dollop of sour cream that made it unattractive to me. I refused to taste it until I was in my twenties. It's been a favorite of mine ever since. If you've never ventured a taste, I hope you will try this recipe.

2 large onions, sliced thin	6 cups water or bouillon
1 tablespoon oil	2 teaspoons salt
1 bunch fresh beets with leaves	½ teaspoon thyme
2 cups shredded cabbage (about	1 bay leaf
½ cabbage head)	Fresh-ground pepper to taste
Juice of 1 fresh lemon	Low-fat sour cream

1. In a large covered kettle, sauté the onions in the oil over low heat until translucent.
2. Pare, clean, and shred the beets in a food processor.
3. Discard the leaf stems, wash the leaves well, and chop.
4. Add all ingredients except sour cream to the onions and bring to a boil.
5. Lower the heat, cover, and simmer for about 45 minutes until beets and cabbage are tender.
6. Stir well, chill, and serve with a dollop of sour cream on each bowlful.

This is a very hearty soup. If you like it thinner, add more water or bouillon and correct the seasonings. ✤

10 servings.

Gazpacho Primo

I think gazpacho takes first place among all cold soups on a hot summer's day. In fact, I like it all year round. This one has plenty of zip and tang, but only a fraction of the oil found in traditional recipes. The puree of half the vegetables gives the soup body, while the chopped remainder gives it a crunchy texture. For interesting body and texture you can use this technique with just about any soup made with vegetables or beans.

1 medium onion, peeled and chopped
3 to 4 cloves garlic, finely minced or crushed
1 tablespoon olive oil
1 large cucumber, peeled, halved lengthwise, and cored to remove seeds, divided
2 large tomatoes, divided
1 green pepper, halved and seeded, divided
3 cups tomato juice, divided
⅓ cup lemon juice
¼ teaspoon hot pepper sauce (Tabasco) or ¼ teaspoon cayenne
¼ teaspoon salt, if desired
⅛ teaspoon fresh-ground black pepper to taste
Croutons for garnish (optional)

1. In a small skillet, sauté onion and garlic in the oil until translucent.
2. In a blender or food processor, combine half the cucumber, 1 tomato, half the green pepper, and 1 cup of the tomato juice.
3. Puree the ingredients at high speed.
4. Chop the remaining cucumber, tomato, and green pepper. Then place them in a bowl, cover, and refrigerate until serving time.
5. Pour the puree into a large serving bowl or tureen, and add the remaining 2 cups of tomato juice and the lemon juice, pepper sauce or cayenne, salt, pepper, and garlic/onion mixture.
6. Refrigerate the gazpacho, covered, for at least 2 hours.
7. Just before serving, add the reserved chopped vegetables.
8. Check the seasonings.
9. Serve the gazpacho with croutons, if desired. ↩

6 servings.

Salad Dressings

Because it is such a good idea to eat about half of all your vegetables in their fresh, raw state, I think it's very important for you to find one or more salad dressings that you really like. And I mean salad dressings that will make eating salads just as enjoyable for you as the foods you most look forward to. At the same time, it's important not to overdo the fat!

Because of the increased interest in lowering fat in the diet, supermarket shelves are loaded with low-fat and no-fat versions of different salad dressings. If you have found one you like, there is no reason to change. But I haven't.

I don't think anything can rival a fresh, homemade dressing, blended exactly to your own tastes. And I like to start with a "full-blooded" dressing, that is, one without water added (which is the way reduced-fat versions are often made). But what about that fat content? On small dinner salads, I think you will find that all it takes is about a teaspoonful to entirely coat the fresh vegetables and give them the flavor and smooth surface texture that make them appealing. However, if you prefer a lower-fat version of any oil-and-vinegar or oil-and-lemon-juice dressing, just add an amount of water equal to $\frac{1}{3}$ the total of oil and vinegar (or lemon juice) and shake well before using.

When eating out, one way to keep the fat at a minimum in full-fat dressings is to have them served on the side, and just dip the tines of your fork before spearing your salad vegetables (something you can always do with other sauces).

Of course, not all salads are made with fresh raw vegetables and eaten cold. You will find a selection of my favorite salads, including some with cooked or partially cooked ingredients, in this section.

Basic Vinaigrette
↔

Traditional vinaigrette dressings start with oil and vinegar, to which are added things like garlic, onions, parsley, and other herbs and flavorings. There is almost no end to the possibilities. This is a basic version, followed by some variations on the theme.

2 tablespoons olive oil
$\frac{1}{4}$ teaspoon salt
$\frac{1}{2}$ teaspoon dried basil

$\frac{1}{4}$ teaspoon dried mustard
1 tablespoon wine vinegar

Whisk oil with all ingredients except vinegar. Add vinegar and whisk again. ✧

Makes 3 tablespoons; serving size is 1 tablespoon.

Garlic Vinaigrette
✧

This is a dressed-up, nippy version of a vinaigrette. It can be made with lemon juice in place of the vinegar, which gives it an entirely different character, and in which case it might better be called a "garlic lemonette." This is, in fact, the way I like it with the Roasted Onion Salad (page 107).

4 cloves garlic	½ teaspoon salt
2 fresh shallots	½ teaspoon fresh-ground black
¼ cup chopped fresh parsley	pepper
½ teaspoon dried crushed red	2 tablespoons white wine vinegar
pepper	⅔ cup olive oil

1. Using the knife blade in your food processor, add the garlic and shallots and pulse 3 or 4 times.
2. Add the parsley and the next 4 ingredients; process 20 seconds, stopping once to scrape down the sides.
3. Pour the olive oil through the food chute in a slow, steady stream with the processor running; process until blended. ✧

Makes 1 cup; serving size is 1 tablespoon.

Lemon and Garlic Dressing
✧

This is a simple and typical eastern Mediterranean salad dressing. It can be used to dress fresh greens, but I include it because it is especially enjoyable as a dressing for steamed or microwaved fresh vegetables.

1 garlic clove, crushed	3 tablespoons extra-virgin olive oil
¼ teaspoon salt	Fresh-ground black pepper to
1 tablespoon fresh lemon juice	taste

1. In a clean dry salad bowl mash the garlic and salt with a spoon to make a smooth paste.

2. Add the lemon juice, stir until the salt is dissolved, then add the olive oil and pepper and mix well.
3. Toss with or drizzle over greens just before serving. ✎

Makes about 4 tablespoons; serving size is 1 tablespoon.

Creamy Tofu Dressing
✎

When my wife, Enid, said she was going to make a tofu dressing, I can't say I was overly excited. Once again, the versatility of tofu showed itself in the delightful, creamy texture it added to the flavor of the other ingredients. When you are looking for a richer style of dressing, try this one.

½ pound firm tofu
2 tablespoons fresh lemon juice
2 tablespoons olive oil
1 tablespoon soy sauce

1 clove garlic, crushed
¼ teaspoon dill weed
¼ teaspoon chili powder

1. Cut the tofu into chunks.
2. Mix the tofu with the other ingredients.
3. Puree all in a blender or food processor, a little at a time, until smooth. ✎

Makes 1 cup; serving size is 1 tablespoon.

Salads

A salad can be one of the most attractive and healthful meals or side dishes to grace your dining table. While it's certainly healthful and refreshing to clear the palette with a mixed green salad, if you think "Cancer Prevention Good Health" and add at least 3 different-colored vegetables to your salads, you will be going a long way toward including hundreds of members of the different families of phytochemicals that are so good for you.

I have included a large variety of salads in this section—some based entirely on vegetables, others made with pasta and different grains, and still others with fish or chicken.

Broccoli Salad

⤫

If you are one of those persons for whom fresh broccoli has an off-putting, grating feel when you bite into it, I think you will find that brief cooking in the microwave will change all that yet leave enough crunch to give this vegetable exactly the right texture. Once you try it, you may want to include briefly microwaved broccoli (or cauliflower) in many of your salads. (The brief cooking helps release some of broccoli's most healthful phytochemicals.)

3 cups broccoli flowerets   Ground pepper to taste
¼ cup water   1 small onion, chopped
2 tablespoons mayonnaise   ½ cup sunflower kernels
1 tablespoon fresh lemon juice   ½ cup raisins
2 tablespoons nonfat yogurt   ½ cup sliced mushrooms
¼ teaspoon chili powder

1. In a microwave, cook the broccoli with the water, covered, on high, for 3 minutes. Drain well.
2. In a small bowl combine the mayonnaise, lemon juice, yogurt, chili powder, and pepper.
3. Put the broccoli and remaining ingredients in a bowl, add the mayonnaise/yogurt mixture, and stir well.
4. Chill.

8 servings.

Note: Instead of mushrooms, you can use ½ cup diced carrots cooked along with the broccoli for 3 minutes. And toasted pine nuts can be substituted for the sunflower kernels (with the addition of ¼ teaspoon of salt). ⤫

Cabbage, Carrot, Green Pepper, and Raisin Salad

⤫

The crunch of the vegetables combined with the sweetness of the raisins and the tangy dressing makes for a refreshing salad.

1 pound cabbage, shredded
2 medium carrots, sliced in thin
  strips
1 green pepper, sliced in thin
  strips
3 tablespoons raisins
4 tablespoons olive oil

2 tablespoons fresh lemon juice
2 teaspoons white wine vinegar
2 teaspoons Dijon mustard
1 teaspoon salt
2 teaspoons poppy seeds
1 teaspoon celery seed
Ground pepper to taste

1. Combine the first 4 ingredients in a large bowl.
2. In another bowl whisk the remaining ingredients and fold into the vegetable mixture.
3. Taste to correct the seasoning.
4. Cover and refrigerate for several hours. ↩

8 servings.

Roasted Onion Salad
↩

This is one of the most popular salads at our dinner parties. We serve it with the "lemonette" version of our Garlic Vinaigrette.

4 medium onions, unpeeled and cut into ½-inch-thick slices
2 tablespoons olive oil and 2 tablespoons lemon juice, blended
8 cups mixed baby lettuce
½ cup walnuts, toasted
2 ounces (4 tablespoons) blue cheese, crumbled
Garlic Vinaigrette (page 104; use lemon juice instead of vinegar)

1. Arrange the onion slices in a lightly greased roasting pan.
2. Drizzle evenly with the olive oil/lemon juice mixture.
3. Bake at 500 degrees for 10 minutes or until the onion slices are lightly charred.
4. Cool the onions, then remove and discard the outer skin. Set aside.
5. Combine lettuce, walnuts, and blue cheese; toss gently.
6. Top with the roasted onion slices.
7. Drizzle with Garlic Vinaigrette. ↩

8 servings.

Main-Course Greek Salad

⊷

This is one of my personal favorites. I make a whole meal out of it by pouring a serving over a big bowl of chopped greens. Try it along with some whole-grain pita bread. It's also one of my favorites when I'm eating out in any Greek restaurant. Often I like it as my main course, and if the restaurant doesn't offer it that way on the menu, I just ask if they will make me one special. Since it's so easy to do, the salad chefs are always glad to oblige. I think they all like making attractive salads as much as I do.

20 Greek or other black olives, pitted and halved
2½ teaspoons capers
1 bunch radishes, chopped (about 10)
1 bunch chives (about ¼ cup)
1 peeled cucumber, scored with fork tines, then halved, seeded, and
    cut in chunks
4 fresh Italian plum tomatoes, cut in chunks
⅛ pound feta cheese, cubed
1 tablespoon olive oil
Juice of ½ fresh lemon
1 teaspoon dried oregano
Black pepper to taste

1. Combine all ingredients except the oil, lemon juice, oregano, and pepper in a large bowl.
2. Whisk the last four ingredients and pour over the salad. Toss to coat, then chill. ⊷

6 servings.

Shredded Cabbage and Carrot Salad

3 cups shredded cabbage (about ½ a large head)
2 carrots, shredded (about 1 cup)
2 tablespoons mayonnaise
2 tablespoons nonfat yogurt
1 tablespoon prepared mustard

½ teaspoon salt
¼ teaspoon garlic powder
¼ teaspoon celery seed
¼ teaspoon crushed red pepper or ground black pepper to taste
1 tablespoon lemon juice

Mix all and chill before serving.

6 servings.

Three-Bean Salad

This is an old favorite that can serve as a side dish on just about any menu. It's great for cookouts and potluck dinners. I often eat any leftovers for lunch the next day, with a chunk of whole-grain bread or crackers.

1 Bermuda or Vidalia onion, sliced thin
1 green bell pepper, diced
2 15-ounce cans cut green beans
2 15-ounce cans cut wax beans
2 15-ounce cans pinto or kidney beans
½ teaspoon garlic powder

1 cup olive oil
½ cup vinegar
½ teaspoon crushed red pepper (optional)
¼ teaspoon ground black pepper
1 teaspoon oregano
2 teaspoons salt

Combine all ingredients in a large bowl and refrigerate overnight. Stir before serving.

8 servings.

Cucumber/Cabbage/Tomato Salad

1 cup shredded cabbage
1 small cucumber, peeled and
   coarsely chopped
1 tomato, coarsely chopped
½ 7-ounce jar hearts of palm or
   artichokes, drained and cubed

½ teaspoon basil
¼ teaspoon salt
1 tablespoon olive oil
1 teaspoon lemon juice
¼ Vidalia or Bermuda onion,
   chopped fine

Combine all in a large bowl and serve. ✌

4 servings.

Rainbow Salad

The different colors among the seven layers in this salad make it look even more beautiful than a seven-layer cake as you view it in a large clear glass bowl. Besides the colors of its somewhat unusual mix of ingredients, it has a rich yet tangy taste that will have guests coming back for seconds. The shredding, dicing, chopping, and toasting take a little time, so do these jobs the night before you plan to serve the salad. The next morning, prepare the dressing, assemble the salad, and refrigerate.

SALAD
3 cups shredded cabbage, green or red
1 cup green or red bell peppers, diced
15-ounce can kernel corn, drained (about 1½ cups)
1 cup shredded carrots
2 cups seedless red or green grapes

DRESSING
½ cup low-fat cottage cheese
2 tablespoons fresh parsley,
   chopped
2 tablespoons mayonnaise
½ teaspoon salt
¼ teaspoon garlic powder
⅛ teaspoon cayenne (optional)
½ cup nonfat plain yogurt

TOPPING
2 tablespoons pine nuts, toasted
2 tablespoons Grape-Nuts

1. Prepare dressing in a food processor or blender by pureeing the cottage cheese with the next 4 ingredients, and cayenne if desired, until smooth.
2. Mix in the yogurt and set aside.
3. Place the cabbage in a 3-inch or taller clear glass bowl (at least 7 inches in diameter, about a 2-quart size) and cover with half the dressing.
4. Layer on the peppers, corn, carrots, and grapes. Cover with the remainder of the dressing.
5. Combine the ingredients for the topping and sprinkle on top.
6. Refrigerate for at least 2 hours—longer is better. ⊹

8 servings.

Pickled Beets
⊹

Pickled beets make a nice counterbalance when served with a richly or thickly flavored main course.

15-ounce can cut beets, drained, reserving ½ cup of juice	2 tablespoons sugar
1 small onion, sliced thin	½ teaspoon salt
½ bell pepper, diced	¼ cup vinegar
¼ cup sliced water chestnuts, rinsed and drained	2 whole cloves
	1 small bay leaf
	3 peppercorns

1. Place the drained beets in a wide-mouthed jar with a lid.
2. Put the remaining ingredients, including the reserved beet juice, in a small saucepan and bring to a boil.
3. Lower the heat and simmer for 1 minute.
4. Remove the mixture from the burner and let it cool several minutes. Pour over the beets.
5. Cover and chill, shaking gently to mix now and then. ⊹

6 servings.

Eggplant Salad

The recipe for this salad has its origin in Catalonia, Spain. The vegetables are cooked first, but served cold mixed with a very flavorful vinaigrette dressing. Once you try it, you may want to use this dressing on other salads as well.

1 large onion, unpeeled
2 red bell peppers
1 eggplant, about 1 pound, cut in half lengthwise
1 medium tomato, cut in ½-inch pieces
2 tablespoons olive oil
1 tablespoon vinegar
1 tablespoon fresh lemon juice
¼ teaspoon Dijon mustard
2 cloves garlic, crushed
1 tablespoon minced fresh parsley

1 teaspoon fresh minced tarragon (or ¼ teaspoon dried)
1 teaspoon fresh minced sage (or ¼ teaspoon dried)
1 tablespoon fresh minced chives (or 1 teaspoon dried)
1 teaspoon dried basil
1 teaspoon salt
1 teaspoon chili powder
Fresh-ground black pepper to taste

1. Preheat oven to 375 degrees.
2. Place onion, peppers, and eggplant halves (skin side up) in an un-oiled baking pan. Roast for 17 minutes.
3. Turn the onion and peppers and roast for 17 minutes more. Let cool.
4. Peel these vegetables and seed the peppers.
5. Cut the onion (remove outer skin), peppers, and eggplant into ½-inch pieces. Refrigerate with the tomato pieces until ready to serve.
6. In a small bowl mix the oil, vinegar, lemon juice, mustard, garlic, herbs, salt, chili powder, and pepper with a whisk or fork. (This can be done in advance and refrigerated.)
7. About 1 hour before serving, mix the vegetables gently with the herb/oil mixture. Serve on pita bread. ↩

6 servings.

Tarragon Chicken Salad with Vermicelli

This is a great way to use leftover poultry. If you start with fresh, you can cook it first in the microwave. And you can even use canned, 98%-fat-free white meat of chicken in a pinch. In the mayonnaise dressing we cut the fat by substituting nonfat yogurt for part of the mayonnaise (I like the proportions at about fifty-fifty). The yogurt adds tartness, while the mayonnaise preserves a rich creamy flavor and texture.

8 ounces dry vermicelli, broken in half (or smaller, if desired)
2 cups cooked, skinless chicken, cut in bite-size chunks
1 cup artichoke hearts, chopped
2 tablespoons nonfat yogurt
2 tablespoons mayonnaise
2 teaspoons prepared mustard
A couple of splashes of rice wine vinegar (or other vinegar of your choice)
1 bunch chopped chives (about ¼ cup)
1 teaspoon dried parsley
½ ounce fresh tarragon, chopped coarsely
8 to 10 inches of anchovy paste
Salt to taste
Fresh-ground black pepper to taste

1. Cook the vermicelli al dente according to the package directions. Drain well, rinse with hot water, and let cool.
2. Combine the remaining ingredients in a large bowl, mixing well. The anchovy paste comes in a squeeze tube. Just squeeze out 8 to 10 inches right into the bowl, to taste.
3. Add the cooled pasta and mix well.
4. Serve immediately or chill first. ↝

8 servings.

Pasta Salad

While this salad is designed primarily to be eaten chilled, it tastes great eaten immediately after mixing with the fresh vegetables.

½ pound whole-wheat seashell pasta (about 2½ cups)
About 2 quarts water to cook pasta
1 teaspoon salt for the water
½ pint cherry tomatoes, halved
1 cucumber, peeled, seeded, and cut in bite-size chunks
2 scallions, chopped
½ green pepper, diced

3 tablespoons mayonnaise
3 tablespoons nonfat plain yogurt
1 tablespoon prepared mustard
1 teaspoon garlic powder
1 tablespoon fresh basil, chopped (or 1 teaspoon dried)
½ teaspoon chili powder
1 teaspoon salt
Pepper to taste

1. Bring about 2 quarts of water to a boil in a large saucepan and add the teaspoon of salt.
2. Add the pasta slowly so that the water doesn't stop boiling.
3. Cook over medium heat, stirring occasionally, for about 10 minutes or until pasta is al dente.
4. Drain and place in a large bowl.
5. Add the vegetables and toss.
6. In a separate small bowl, mix the remainder of the ingredients together and then pour over the pasta mixture. Toss well to coat.
7. Chill and serve. ✎

8 servings.

Greek Couscous Salad

Although this dish is customarily chilled before eating, it's good warm, too.

1 cup couscous
1½ cups chicken bouillon
½ cup chopped fresh parsley
3 tablespoons olive oil
1 tablespoon freshly squeezed
  lemon juice
½ teaspoon dried mint
½ teaspoon dried basil
½ teaspoon dried oregano

1 teaspoon dried thyme
½ teaspoon salt (or more to
  taste)
Ground black pepper to taste
2 large tomatoes, chopped
3 tablespoons crumbled feta
  cheese
Sliced cucumber for garnish

1. Place the couscous in a large bowl.
2. Bring the chicken bouillon to a boil and pour over the couscous. Stir and let sit for about 15 minutes until all the liquid has been absorbed. Then fluff with a fork and set aside.
3. In a medium-sized bowl combine the parsley, oil, lemon juice, and spices. Whisk until smooth.
4. Add the tomatoes and feta cheese, stir, and pour over the couscous. Stir to combine; taste and adjust the seasonings.
5. Chill for at least 30 minutes. Garnish with cucumbers and serve. ✎

8 servings.

Chicken, Rice, and Artichoke Salad

This is a good main dish at either lunch or supper. It makes for a colorful as well as healthful plate accompanied by winter squash or carrots.

DRESSING
2 tablespoons red wine
  vinegar
2 scallions, chopped
1 tablespoon grated fresh ginger
  (or 1 teaspoon dried)

2 teaspoons prepared Dijon
  mustard
¼ teaspoon salt
Pepper to taste
4 tablespoons olive oil

15-ounce can artichoke hearts, rinsed, patted dry, and diced

2 cups cooked brown rice

2 5-ounce cans 98%-fat-free chicken packed in broth

2 tablespoons ketchup

1 small red bell pepper, diced

1 scallion, thinly sliced

¼ teaspoon salt

¼ teaspoon each dried tarragon, sage, and chives

Pepper to taste

Romaine lettuce

Parsley for garnish (optional)

1. In a small bowl blend all of the dressing ingredients, adding the olive oil last and whisking well.
2. In a large mixing bowl combine the salad ingredients except for the lettuce and parsley.
3. Whisk the dressing again and pour over the salad, stirring to combine.
4. Serve on beds of coarsely torn Romaine lettuce or lettuce leaves, and garnish with parsley if desired. ❧

12 servings.

Mexican Quinoa Salad

❧

Quinoa is really a seed from a pigweed grown in the high Andes Mountains. It can be found in health-food stores and will make a tasty and nutritious addition to your salad repertoire in combination with a variety of different vegetables and beans.

2 tablespoons plus 1 teaspoon olive oil, divided

½ cup quinoa, rinsed in cold water and drained

1 cup vegetable or chicken bouillon

¼ teaspoon dried tarragon

1 teaspoon salt

1½ tablespoons fresh lime juice

Ground black pepper to taste

1 cup canned drained black beans

1 cup frozen corn kernels, defrosted

1 small red bell pepper, cut in thin strips

1 tomato, chopped

2 scallions, chopped

½ teaspoon dried basil

1 teaspoon dried cilantro

2 tablespoons chopped fresh parsley

½ teaspoon chili powder

1. Heat 1 teaspoon of the oil in a small saucepan.
2. Add the quinoa and cook over low heat, stirring, for 5 minutes.
3. Stir in the bouillon, tarragon, and salt and bring to a boil. Then lower the heat and simmer, covered, for 15 minutes. Fluff with a fork and set aside.
4. In a large bowl, whisk the remaining oil with the lime juice and pepper.
5. Stir in all the rest of the vegetables and spices.
6. Add the quinoa and stir.
7. Taste and adjust the seasonings.
8. Chill for at least 1 hour, then let it come to room temperature and serve. ✺

8 servings.

Tuna with Chickpeas
✺

This is a very satisfying main-dish dinner salad, originating in Greece. It's one of my favorite leftover dishes for lunch.

15-ounce can chickpeas, drained
2 6-ounce cans tuna packed in
　water, drained
4 scallions, chopped
1 stalk celery, chopped
2 tablespoons olive oil
2 garlic cloves, crushed
Grated rind of ½ lemon
1 tablespoon freshly squeezed
　lemon juice

3 tablespoons chopped parsley
　(plus additional leaves for
　optional garnish)
1 teaspoon dried dill
½ teaspoon salt
Fresh-ground black pepper to
　taste
¼ teaspoon dried mustard

1. Place the drained chickpeas and tuna in a medium-sized bowl and stir in the scallions and celery.
2. In another bowl combine all the other ingredients and whisk to blend.
3. Stir this dressing into the tuna mixture.
4. Cover and chill for several hours before serving, garnished with parsley if desired. ✺

4 servings.

Artichoke and Crab-Meat Salad

꩜

Another Greek-style salad that you can whip up on the spur of the moment. We have served this on occasion as an appetizer.

1 cup diced artichoke hearts   1 tablespoon mayonnaise
6½-ounce can crabmeat   1 teaspoon lemon juice
¼ cup chopped ripe olives   Salt and pepper to taste

Combine all ingredients and serve on toast. ꩜

4 servings.

Meat

If you prefer to include red meat in your diet yet wish to minimize the health risks, I suggest you use only the leanest cuts. With beef, this means flank steak or London broil, and eye of round and top round, well trimmed, for roasts. The leanest cut of pork is the tenderloin. These cuts have less than a quarter the amount of fat found in rib-eye steaks, chuck roasts, and regular pork chops.

I include two marinades for tenderizing and seasoning flank steak and London broil, and a recipe for a particularly well-seasoned pork tenderloin roast. Try them—if you have been eating fattier cuts of meat, with these recipes you won't miss them.

Steak Marinade

꩜

These marinades prepare lean steak cuts for pan or oven broiling. Both the wine and soy sauce have a tenderizing effect, so marinate overnight in the refrigerator, in a large covered bowl or plastic bag. Turn the meat once or twice while it is marinating, to be sure all of it has been well covered.

I include oil in these marinades as an option because it helps the marinade adhere to the meat and gives the meat a somewhat better texture. It's not absolutely necessary, but I used to include it when I made these steaks in the past. And, whether or not you decide to use some oil, if you puncture the meat with the tines of a fork and then rub it lightly with a bit of flour, the marinade will be absorbed more fully into the flesh, thereby increasing both the flavor and the tenderizing effect.

The amounts of marinade in these recipes will do nicely for 2 pounds of meat, which, after being reduced by about 25 percent during broiling, will yield 1½ pounds, or 4 large servings (that is, double size, 6 ounces each).

BASIC MARINADE

1 teaspoon olive oil (optional)
½ cup dry red wine (use white wine for light-colored meats)
¼ teaspoon Herb Salt (page 183)

1 bay leaf
1 teaspoon dried chives
1 small onion, minced

ORIENTAL MARINADE

1 teaspoon olive oil (optional)
¼ cup tamari sauce or soy sauce
¼ cup dry red wine
4 cloves garlic, minced
4 scallions, minced

6 whole peppercorns
⅛ teaspoon ground coriander
1-inch cube fresh ginger, peeled and grated or minced

Flank steaks and London broil are most tender when sliced thin, against the grain, on the bias. ✎

Roast Pork Tenderloin

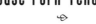

Pork tenderloin is about the easiest cut of pork to prepare, and it does make a memorable roast. One and a half pounds of meat will reduce in cooking and yield about 6 Food-Pyramid-size servings, 3 ounces each. Pork tenderloin usually comes packaged in two separate small strips. Tie them together (one on top of the other) with several separate strands of butcher's twine, about 2 inches between ties.

½ teaspoon thyme
½ teaspoon marjoram
½ teaspoon sage
½ teaspoon garlic powder
½ teaspoon onion powder
½ teaspoon ground ginger

Fresh-ground black pepper to taste
2 tablespoons tamari or soy sauce
1 tablespoon Worcestershire sauce
1½ pounds pork roast

1. Place all dry ingredients in a small bowl.
2. Add the soy sauce and Worcestershire sauce and mix well.
3. Spread the mixture evenly over the meat and allow it to marinate for an hour or two in the refrigerator.
4. Roast at 350 degrees until the internal temperature reaches 170°F (about 40–45 minutes).
5. To serve, slice in ¼-inch pieces and arrange on a platter surrounded by rice or vegetables.

6 3-ounce servings.

VARIATIONS

1. If you wish, you can add 1 teaspoon of olive oil to the marinade. The oil helps the marinade stick to the meat, and since some of the marinade cooks away during roasting and some sticks to the pan, you will add only a couple of grams of fat to the entire roast. To increase tenderness and flavor, puncture the meat with the tines of a fork and coat very lightly with flour before applying the marinade.
2. Company version: Use 4 cloves of garlic (minced), 3 green onions (chopped), and a 1-inch piece of ginger (minced) in place of the dry ingredients.
3. When you are in a hurry, simply rub the meat with 2 tablespoons of Dijon mustard and 2 cloves of garlic (minced) before roasting. ✎

Fish

When I question people who care little for fish, I usually find they don't know how to prepare it. The first rule for preparing excellent fish dishes is DON'T OVERCOOK THEM. While there is a rather big window for cooking fatty fish, such as salmon, where several extra minutes in the oven or on the grill will not ruin them, fish with little fat (cod, flounder, sole, haddock, halibut) reach their best flavor and texture and maintain them for only a couple of minutes during the cooking process. You must catch them at their best! They need careful watching until you know exactly how long and at what temperature to cook them in your oven or on your grill or stove-top burner. I say this because stove ovens and burners can vary considerably even when set at similar temperatures. Once you have experimented with your stove, you can be more relaxed.

And when people say they are not fond of fish, they have usually not experimented with the various ways of preparing them. Fish is a versatile food; you can broil, steam, bake, grill, and poach. Fish lends itself to both the simplest methods of preparation and rather complex combinations of flavors. Try out my Baked Fish Fillets to test a fail-safe method for baking fish. This recipe will show you how easy it is to prepare lean fish fillets, and you will see how long it takes in your oven. Then, for comparison, try out the same recipe using a fatty fish, such as salmon (this appears as part of the same recipe, as a variation). Finally, I include a few recipes to illustrate more complex combinations, using different vegetables and seasonings, yielding different flavors.

Baked Fish Fillets

᠂ᢒ

This is one of the simplest ways to prepare fish and one of the most satisfying.

1½ pounds lean fish fillets (sole, flounder, perch)	Salt and pepper to taste Garlic and onion powder to taste (optional)
1 tablespoon olive oil	
1 teaspoon lemon juice	

1. Preheat oven to 375 degrees.
2. Pour the oil and lemon juice onto a foil-lined baking pan.
3. Swish the fish around in the liquid on both sides.
4. Sprinkle with salt and pepper, and garlic and onion powder if desired.
5. Bake 8 to 12 minutes uncovered on an oven shelf just above the middle of your oven (possibly the second level below the grilling shelf in an electric oven).
6. Be sure to test at 8 minutes and frequently thereafter. Fish is done when it flakes easily with a fork, and is still moist.

4 servings.

VARIATION

Make the same recipe with a fatty fish, such as salmon. Salmon fillets may take 10 to 15 minutes, while steaks an inch in thickness can take 15 to 20 minutes. Until you know your oven, test frequently for doneness. Salmon is done when there is still a little streak of pinkness in the center, and the fish is moist and flakes easily with a fork. ᠂ᢒ

Baked Swordfish

This is similar to the method used in the previous recipe, but adds a step, with crushed rosemary and flour, that changes the character considerably.

1½ to 1¾ pounds swordfish	2 teaspoons dried rosemary, crushed
1 tablespoon olive oil	Flour
1 teaspoon lemon juice	Salt and pepper to taste

1. Combine oil and lemon juice in a foil-lined baking pan.
2. Put rosemary in mortar and crush with pestle to release aroma and flavor.
3. Press rosemary onto both sides of fish.
4. Sprinkle with flour and rub that into both sides of fish.
5. Put the fish in the pan and rub both sides of it into the oil/lemon juice mixture.
6. Add salt and pepper to taste.
7. Bake at 350 degrees for 15 minutes, then raise the heat to 375 degrees and bake for 5 minutes longer. Test for doneness. ↬

4 servings.

Teriyaki Salmon

This is my favorite recipe for salmon fillets. You can use salmon steaks, but they will not be as tender. I like salmon baked only to the point where there is still a tiny streak of pink in the center and the flesh is moist and flaky. Try it this way before you cook it any longer!

1½ pounds salmon fillets (or 4 steaks, about 6 ounces each)
1 tablespoon olive oil
1 teaspoon lemon juice
1 tablespoon tamari (or soy) sauce
1 teaspoon Worcestershire sauce
1-inch piece of fresh ginger, minced (or ½ teaspoon ground ginger)
1 clove garlic, minced (or ½ teaspoon garlic powder), optional
Fresh-ground black pepper to taste
Paprika

1. Preheat oven to 375 degrees.
2. Spread liquid ingredients in a shallow, foil-lined baking dish.
3. Sprinkle in the fresh ginger, garlic (optional), and black pepper and mix with the liquid.
4. Swish both sides of the fish around in the mixture.
5. Sprinkle fish lightly with paprika (if using fillets, lay skin side down in the pan).
6. Place on an oven shelf about three-quarters of the way up.
7. Bake for 10 to 15 minutes, testing for doneness. Thicker pieces of fish may take up to 20 minutes. ✐

4 servings.

Orange Roughy with Spinach
✐

Orange roughy is a medium-fatty fish that can be prepared as specified in Baked Fish Fillets, but it also lends itself to a rich-tasting Florentine combination. You can use any lean to medium-fatty fillets in this recipe.

1½ pounds orange roughy fillets (2 fillets)
8 ounces fresh spinach
2 teaspoons olive oil
2 tablespoons soy sauce
2 teaspoons Worcestershire sauce

1 medium onion, sliced thinly
1 medium tomato, sliced thinly
2 tablespoons grated Parmesan
Fresh-ground black pepper to taste

1. Preheat oven to 375 degrees.
2. Line a 3-inch-deep baking pan with half the spinach.
3. Place fish on top.
4. Combine olive oil with soy sauce and Worcestershire and drizzle over fish.
5. Partially cook the onion (5 minutes on high in the microwave).
6. Spread the onion and tomato slices over the fish.
7. Sprinkle Parmesan and pepper on top and spread the remaining spinach on top of that.
8. Cover lightly with aluminum foil and bake 20–25 minutes or until fish flakes easily with a fork. ✐

4 servings.

Seafood Stove-Top Casserole

·ᴥ·

You can serve this dish as is, in a bowl with great hunks of bread on the side, or pour it over brown rice. It's one fish dish that doesn't suffer from being reheated and served as a leftover. And instead of limiting yourself to just one kind of fish in this recipe, try a mix.

2 cups fish stock or light chicken bouillon
1 cup dry white wine
1 bay leaf
1 cup sliced fresh mushrooms
2 red bell peppers, sliced into strips
1 tablespoon dried parsley (or ⅓ cup fresh parsley, minced)
Fresh-ground black pepper to taste
4 cups cooked lobster, crab, scallops, or monkfish, cut into chunks
2 eggs
2 teaspoons cayenne pepper
1 tablespoon dry mustard
4 pimiento strips (optional)

1. Bring the stock and wine to a boil in a large saucepan.
2. Add the bay leaf, mushrooms, sliced peppers, parsley, and black pepper to the stock, reduce the heat, and let simmer for about 5 to 10 minutes, until the vegetables are just tender. Add the seafood, and simmer 5 minutes more.
3. In the meantime, blend the eggs, cayenne pepper, and dry mustard together. Add to the seafood, and let simmer for a couple more minutes.
4. Serve garnished with pimiento strips, if desired. ·ᴥ·

8 servings.

Poultry

While most experts are encouraging the use of chicken and other poultry as a garnish or condiment in combination with grains and vegetables, they still feel that chicken, as well as fish, can play a healthful role as a main course in your diet. A total of about 6 ounces a day should be your maximum, and there is no need to have chicken or fish every day.

Because ground turkey has been touted as a good substitute for ground beef by many nutritionists, I want to warn you that regular ground turkey is just as full of fat as regular ground beef. You should ask for extra lean when purchasing fresh ground turkey at your supermarket, and read the labels carefully on the national brands. They can be misleading. For example, one popular brand claims "40% less fat than regular ground beef." That assumes regular ground beef contains around 24% fat. Their lower-fat version of turkey contains 16 grams of fat per ½-cup serving, which is still about 14% fat. That is definitely not a low-fat product. Look for ground turkey that is less than 10% fat, and preferably less than 5%.

You can make a lean roast chicken by removing the skin before cooking, and, to preserve moisture and add flavor, make a basting sauce with a ½ cup of ketchup, 2 tablespoons of tamari or soy sauce, and 2 ounces of sherry. Coat the chicken well before putting it in the oven, sprinkle with your choice of herbs (and garlic and onion powder if desired), and cover it lightly for about half the cooking time. This is also a simple and quick way to prepare baked chicken pieces. You will find my favorite "oven-fried" recipe on page 129.

For interesting and unusual flavors, mix any one of the garam masalas (page 181) with a bit of oil and tamari (or soy sauce) to make a paste, and coat a whole chicken (or pieces) before roasting or baking.

Broiled Chicken with Yogurt

Chicken legs are used in this recipe, but other chicken pieces work equally well. The yogurt is used not only for flavor but also to tenderize the meat, making it more succulent and juicy. Use the salt sparingly; you can always add more at the table.

12 skinless chicken legs (about 2 pounds)
3 garlic cloves, crushed
¼ teaspoon fresh-ground black pepper, or to taste
Salt to taste
1 teaspoon paprika
1 teaspoon ground cinnamon

½ teaspoon nutmeg
Pinch of cayenne pepper
Freshly squeezed juice of 1 lemon
2 tablespoons olive oil
½ cup nonfat yogurt
Lemon wedges

1. Place the chicken legs in a large, shallow dish.
2. In a medium-sized bowl, combine the garlic, pepper, salt, paprika, cinnamon, nutmeg, cayenne, lemon juice, oil (if white meat is used, double the amount of oil), and yogurt.

3. Pour the marinade over the chicken legs, stirring and turning them to coat evenly. Cover and leave to marinate in the refrigerator for 2–3 hours or overnight.
4. Season the chicken legs again with a little more salt and fresh-ground black pepper (optional).
5. Place the chicken legs on an oiled broiler rack under a preheated broiler and cook for 20–40 minutes or until crisp and golden on the outside and cooked through, turning frequently during cooking.
6. Serve with lemon wedges. ❧

6 servings of 2 legs each.

Curried Chicken and Spinach
❧

This is a spicy way to make chicken and greens. For variety, you can also try one of the garam masala recipes (page 181) in place of the spices suggested here.

BOTTOM LAYER
2 cups coarsely chopped onion (2 large onions)
2 teaspoons minced garlic
2 tablespoons oil and 2 tablespoons water
2 10-ounce packages frozen spinach, thawed and drained
1 teaspoon each salt, ground coriander, and turmeric
½ teaspoon cayenne

1. Cook the onion and garlic in the oil/water mixture until translucent.
2. Combine this mixture with the spinach and spices.
3. Place on the bottom of a lightly oiled 12×8-inch baking dish.

TOP LAYER
6 skinless chicken breast halves
1 tablespoon lime juice
1 tablespoon oil
¼ teaspoon turmeric

1. Place the chicken breasts on the spinach layer.
2. Combine the lime juice, oil, and turmeric and brush on the chicken.
3. Bake, *uncovered,* at 325 degrees for 1 hour, or until done.

RICE
1½ cups brown rice
1 tablespoon oil
3 cups vegetable broth
1 teaspoon salt (optional)
¼ teaspoon each sage, thyme, and rosemary

1. In a saucepan, sauté the rice in the oil for about 2 minutes.
2. Add the vegetable broth and spices.
3. Place in a casserole, *cover,* and bake along with the chicken at 325 degrees for 1 hour. ✈

6 servings.

Oven-Stewed Chicken and Vegetables
✈
This is a rich meal in a casserole, and very easy to prepare.

4 skinless chicken breasts (or 8 thighs)
2 large potatoes, halved lengthwise and sliced ½ inch thick
2 large carrots, in ½-inch slices
1 large onion, in thick slices
4 stalks celery, thinly sliced
1 green bell pepper, in ½-inch slices
2 15-ounce cans tomato sauce
About 2 cups chicken bouillon, to almost cover mixture
½ teaspoon garlic powder
½ teaspoon each thyme and marjoram
Fresh-ground black pepper to taste

1. Wash the chicken breasts and place on the bottom of a 5-quart casserole dish.
2. Spread the vegetables around on top of the chicken breasts.
3. Pour in the tomato sauce and chicken bouillon until the vegetables are just about covered (do not quite cover since the water contained in the vegetables will be released in the casserole).
4. Sprinkle the garlic powder, herbs, and pepper over the mixture and blend into the liquid and vegetables on the surface.
5. Cover and bake in a 350-degree oven for about 1½ to 2 hours, stirring and mixing the ingredients every half hour or so. If you have to leave

your home for any reason during the cooking, you can turn down the heat to 250 degrees and let the casserole simmer for 3 or even 4 hours without stirring and it will be just fine, like most pot roasts or stews. ∽

4 servings.

Roast Poultry, Tandoori Style
∽

Once a year, at Thanksgiving or Christmas, I like to roast a turkey in a style somewhat similar to the Tandoori method. It's the only time that I do something intentionally that has questionable health consequences. I use a covered outdoor grill for cooking over charcoal since I don't have the traditional Indian-style cylindrical clay oven, and I use paprika for coloring, rather than the traditional liquid red food coloring. You can also roast the bird in your indoor oven, if you prefer, since outdoor grilling or smoking should be done only rarely. The seasoning and cooking methods work well with chicken, too, and it takes considerably less time.

1 fresh turkey	½ teaspoon onion powder
1 tablespoon garam masala (see page 181)	Paprika
	1 tablespoon olive oil
½ teaspoon garlic powder	1 teaspoon soy sauce

FOR COOKING ON A COVERED, OUTDOOR GRILL

1. Remove the rack (you will place the poultry on a double sheet of extra-heavy aluminum foil on this rack and place it back in the grill later). Get your grill fire started, and ready to be controlled at a low constant heat. You will have to add pieces of charcoal periodically, to maintain heat for 6 or more hours, for a large turkey.
2. Combine the spices, oil, and soy sauce in a small bowl to make a paste.
3. Rub the paste all over the turkey, pressing lightly into the skin.
4. Make a platter for the turkey out of extra-heavy aluminum foil, with the sides turned up at least 2 inches all around to catch juices, and place on the grill rack.
5. Move the turkey onto the platter, and then sprinkle liberally with extra paprika.
6. Place a meat thermometer in the thickest part of the breast, well into the flesh, but not touching any bone.
7. Take another sheet of aluminum foil and make a cover for the turkey

with a slit in it for the thermometer to poke through and cover the poultry lightly with it.

8. Place in the grill, cover the grill, baste occasionally, maintain heat with added charcoal, and roast until done (meat thermometer should read 195°F).

Serving size is 3 ounces.

FOR COOKING IN AN INDOOR GAS OR ELECTRIC OVEN

Follow Steps 2 and 3 above, sprinkle with extra paprika, insert the meat thermometer as in Step 6, cover as in Step 7, and then roast at 350 degrees until the thermometer reaches 195°F. ✑

Oven-Fried Chicken

I have made this recipe on various TV shows to illustrate how to make a great-tasting "oven-fried" version of one of America's favorite foods. The studio staffs make short work of it after the shows.

1 tablespoon vegetable oil	¼ teaspoon salt
1 teaspoon lemon juice	¼ teaspoon fresh-ground black
3 pounds chicken pieces,	pepper
skinned	¼ teaspoon onion powder
About ⅓ cup skim or 1% milk or	¼ teaspoon garlic powder
buttermilk	⅛ teaspoon cayenne pepper
½ cup flour (all purpose, whole	¼ teaspoon marjoram
wheat, or combination)	¼ teaspoon oregano
1½ teaspoons paprika	

1. Combine the oil and lemon juice, and brush each piece of skinned chicken with the mixture.
2. Place the milk in a shallow bowl, and set aside. Combine the flour(s) and seasonings in another bowl, mixing well.
3. Dip the chicken pieces into the milk, coating all sides. Then coat with the flour mixture.
4. Place the chicken "skin" side up in a foil-covered baking pan. Cover loosely with foil, and bake at 350 degrees for 60 minutes. ✑

6 servings.

Casseroles and Main Dishes

I have placed eight of my heartiest, most filling dishes in this section. Several of them illustrate how we use fish or poultry as a complement to grains and vegetables. Except for the Onion Quiche, most of these dishes need just a small dinner salad to round out the meal. With the Onion Quiche, which is a bit lighter, I'd add both a starchy and non-starchy vegetable.

Tuna Casserole

1 onion, chopped
1 clove garlic, minced
1 tablespoon oil
1 tablespoon chopped fresh
   parsley
1 cup diced fresh tomatoes
   (about 2 tomatoes)
1 teaspoon salt

1 teaspoon sage
½ teaspoon thyme
Fresh-ground pepper to taste
Dash of cayenne (optional)
2 cups cooked brown rice
2 6-ounce cans water-packed
   tuna, drained

1. In a large skillet, sauté the onion and garlic in the oil until translucent.
2. Add parsley, tomatoes, and seasonings and cook, covered, for 10 minutes.
3. Add the rice and tuna, blend well, and turn into a casserole dish.
4. Bake at 350 degrees for about 30 minutes.

6 servings.

Escarole Torte

This is our version of a northern Italian recipe.

1 large head escarole
2 quarts boiling water
2 pounds potatoes (3 large),
   washed and cut into chunks
2 tablespoons olive oil

1 tablespoon butter
¼–½ cup 1% milk
Salt and pepper to taste
½ cup grated Parmesan, divided
1 cup cooked chickpeas

1. Wash the escarole well and push down into the boiling water.
2. Let cook, uncovered, for about 7 minutes.

3. When done, remove the escarole with a slotted spoon and press it against the sides of a sieve to get rid of excess moisture.
4. Coarsely chop it.
5. Meanwhile, using the escarole liquid, boil the potatoes until tender, drain, and, in a large mixing bowl, mash with the olive oil, butter, milk, salt to taste, and ¼ cup of cheese.
6. Add the escarole, chickpeas, and salt and pepper to taste.
7. Place the entire mixture in a large casserole dish and sprinkle with the remaining cheese.
8. Bake at 350 degrees for 20 minutes.

8 servings.

Don't forget to freeze the cooking water for later use in soups and stews. ✎

Southwest Casserole

The ingredients for this colorful casserole are added in layers, rather than mixed.

LAYERS	TOPPING
2 cups cooked brown rice	1 cup nonfat plain yogurt
2 cups cooked, cubed chicken	⅓ cup chopped scallions
½ cup shredded Monterey Jack cheese or cheddar	½ teaspoon salt
4-ounce can chopped chiles, drained	1 teaspoon chili powder
1 pint cherry tomatoes, halved	¼ teaspoon dried oregano (or 1 teaspoon fresh, chopped)
	Ground black pepper to taste
	½ cup shredded Monterey Jack cheese or cheddar

1. Spread the rice in a lightly oiled 3-quart casserole.
2. Add, in layers, the chicken, cheese, chiles, and tomatoes.
3. Mix the topping ingredients and spread over the casserole.
4. Bake at 350 degrees for 30 minutes. ✎

6 servings.

Onion Quiche

When our testers compared quiches made with whole eggs versus those made with just egg whites (using Egg Beaters), the egg whites won out every time.

½ cup stuffing mix or
   breadcrumbs
1 teaspoon butter, melted
4 large onions, sliced thin
2 cloves garlic, crushed
1 tablespoon olive oil
1 cup Egg Beaters (equivalent to
   4 eggs)
1 cup 1% milk

1 tablespoon cornstarch
1 teaspoon salt
¼ teaspoon nutmeg
Ground black pepper to taste
1 tablespoon fresh chopped
   chives (or 1 teaspoon dried)
1 tablespoon nutritional yeast
¼ cup shredded cheddar

1. Lightly oil a pie pan.
2. Crush the stuffing mix or use breadcrumbs and combine with the butter.
3. Press onto the bottom and a short way up the sides of the oiled pie pan.
4. Refrigerate until needed.
5. Braise onions and garlic in the olive oil, partly covered, until onions are translucent.
6. Spread in the pie plate.
7. Whisk the Egg Beaters with the milk, cornstarch, salt, spices, chives, and yeast.
8. Add the cheddar and stir.
9. Pour over the onions and bake at 350 degrees for about 25 minutes or until set in the middle. ↪

6 servings.

Stuffed Winter Squash

⊸

These can be assembled early in the day and baked later.

2 medium or 3 small squash,
   either butternut or acorn
½ pound ground low-fat turkey
1 cup chopped onions
1 cup frozen whole kernel corn,
   defrosted
½ cup minced carrots
½ teaspoon cumin

½ cup V8 juice
4-ounce can chopped green
   chiles, with juice
¾ cup cooked brown rice
½ teaspoon salt
⅛ teaspoon ground black pepper
¼ cup shredded cheddar cheese

1. Cut the squash in half and scoop out the seeds.
2. Put them in microwave-safe casseroles, cut side down, cover with waxed paper, and cook, on high, for about 15 minutes or until squash is tender. (If you don't have a microwave, the squash can be baked in a 350-degree oven, cut side down, in about 1 inch of water until tender.)
3. In a 3-quart saucepan, over medium heat, cook the turkey with the onions, corn, carrots, and cumin until the turkey is cooked through and the onions are tender. Stir while cooking so the turkey gets separated.
4. Then stir in the V8 juice, chiles, rice, salt, and pepper. Heat to boiling and then remove from heat and let stand a few minutes.
5. Stir in the cheese and then fill the squash halves with the mixture.
6. If necessary, you can scoop a bit of the squash out and reserve for another purpose if you need to make more room for the filling.
7. Bake in a 350-degree oven for about 15 minutes, or until hot. ⊸

4 to 6 servings.

Tamale Pie

⊸

TOPPING
1 cup 1% milk
1 tablespoon lemon juice
1 tablespoon oil

1 cup cornmeal
1 teaspoon baking soda
¼ teaspoon salt

1. In a small bowl combine the milk, lemon juice, and oil.
2. In another bowl combine the cornmeal, baking soda, and salt.
3. Add the milk mixture to the dry ingredients and stir until moistened.

FILLING

2 teaspoons oil
2 onions, diced
2 cloves garlic, minced
2 tomatoes, diced
2 15-ounce cans pinto or other
    beans, drained
2 4-ounce cans diced green
    chiles, with juice

½ teaspoon salt
1 teaspoon dried basil
1 teaspoon cumin
½ teaspoon crushed red pepper
    (optional)

1. Heat the oil in a 3-quart saucepan.
2. Add the onions and garlic, cover, and cook on medium-low heat until the onions are translucent.
3. Add the tomatoes and cook about 3 minutes longer.
4. Add the beans, chiles, salt, and spices, raise heat to medium, and bring to a boil. Remove from heat.
5. Mash a few of the beans against the sides of the pan.
6. Transfer to an 8×11×2-inch oblong baking dish.
7. Pour the topping over the beans and bake in a 400-degree oven for 30 minutes. ✏

8 servings.

Monna's White Chili

One comes across great recipes in all sorts of places. Monna Journey is my dental hygienist, and when I mentioned, in the dental chair at a recent visit, that I was in the process of gathering recipes for my new book, this "primo" among all chili recipes was my reward.

1 pound large white beans (such
    as Great Northern)
6 cups water
6 cups chicken broth
2 medium onions, chopped
2 cloves garlic, minced

2 tablespoons olive oil
2 4-ounce cans chopped green
    chiles
2 teaspoons ground cumin
1½ teaspoons oregano
¼ teaspoon cayenne

¼ teaspoon ground cloves
4 cups cooked chicken breasts,
   diced
16-ounce jar of salsa

Shredded part-skim mozzarella
   and low-fat sour cream
   (optional)

1. Soak the beans overnight in the 6 cups of water.
2. Drain, rinse, add the chicken broth, half of the onions, and the garlic, and put in a 6-quart kettle (with lid).
3. Bring to a boil, then lower heat and simmer, covered, until beans are tender (about 3 hours). Stir occasionally and add more water if necessary.
4. In a skillet, sauté the remaining onions in the oil until tender.
5. Add the chiles and the seasonings and mix well.
6. When the beans are tender, add the onion mixture and the chicken.
7. Bring to a boil again, then lower heat, cover, and let simmer for 1 hour.
8. Place in a serving bowl and pour salsa over the top.
9. Top each serving with mozzarella and low-fat sour cream (optional). ✎

8 servings.

Savory Turkey Loaf
✎

The National Turkey Federation provided the inspiration for this recipe. My wife, Enid, was intrigued by the idea of combining turkey and spinach, and then went on to create her own mixture of seasonings.

1 pound lean ground turkey
10-ounce package frozen
   chopped spinach, thawed and
   drained
½ cup stuffing mix
1 small onion, chopped
1 clove garlic, crushed
2½ tablespoons prepared Dijon
   mustard

¼ cup fresh parsley, chopped
¼ teaspoon dried thyme
1 tablespoon ketchup
¼ cup shredded part-skim
   mozzarella
2-ounce jar chopped pimientos,
   drained

1. Preheat oven to 350 degrees.
2. Lightly oil a 9-inch pie pan.
3. In a large bowl, combine all but the last three ingredients.

4. Shape into a loaf, about 4 × 6 inches in size, in the pie pan.
5. Bake the turkey loaf for about 55 minutes.
6. Spread with ketchup and sprinkle on the cheese and pimientos.
7. Bake about 5 minutes longer, until cheese is melted. ❧

4 servings.

Grains and Legumes

Legumes, grains, sprouts, nuts, and seeds are the valuable non-animal sources of protein. At the same time, they are loaded with fiber and other phytochemicals with health-enhancing properties. We use a large variety of different beans—right now, in our pantry, we have small red beans, larger kidney beans, pintos, black and white beans, and soybeans. They are so easy to prepare! All it really takes, in the most simple method of preparation, is 1 cup of dried beans and 2 cups of chicken bouillon. You can soak the beans in advance, or not (although some preliminary soaking is best for soybeans). Sometimes I just wash my beans (except for soys) in hot water, drain, and start the cooking process. If you don't have home-made stock, try a commercial version (I like Wyler's) at half strength—that is, ½ teaspoon per cup of water. You will be surprised at how good this easy recipe tastes.

Beans are sometimes called "whistle berries" because they tend to create a lot of gas in people who are not accustomed to eating them. While countless remedies have been proposed, most of little value, I know of two that can help. First, eat beans more frequently in modest amounts! Your system will develop the intestinal flora that can deal with them, creating very little gas. By "more frequently," I mean a portion three or more times a week. Most people are amazed at the change in the way their systems deal with them. Sometimes people find that only certain varieties make them uncomfortable—for example, pintos or kidneys, but not black beans, or vice versa. It's worth a little experimentation to determine your own system's idiosyncrasies. Second, try the commercial product Beano. At least one study has shown some relief with its use.

Many of our dishes combine grains with legumes and other plant foods. You will find millet, barley, rice, couscous, and other wheat products in the following recipes. But there are many other kinds of grains and many delicious ways to combine them with other plant foods, which you can find in cookbooks that emphasize plant foods.

A Simple Pot of Beans
❧

These beans can be refrigerated after cooking and incorporated into any recipe that calls for beans. The recipe may be multiplied and cooked in larger quantities. The consistency and flavor of these beans are fine without overnight soaking before cooking. The recipe works well with any kind of dried bean, but note that most varieties of dried beans, especially larger ones, require more cooking than the small red beans and may improve with prior soaking.

1 cup small red beans (dry)
3 cups water (or bouillon, and
    omit salt)
1 small onion, chopped
2–3 cloves garlic, chopped
1 teaspoon salt

1 teaspoon olive oil (less if
    desired)
½ teaspoon cayenne or fresh
    chopped jalapeño pepper
    (optional)

1. Rinse the beans, combine with the water or bouillon in a 2-quart saucepan, and bring to a boil.
2. Turn the heat to low, add all the other ingredients, and cook 1 hour, covered, then stir.
3. Add more water as necessary.
4. Cook another hour on low and test for doneness (it may take longer). When done, turn heat off and allow beans to cool slowly in the pot on the stove. They'll be just right for eating after about an hour.

6 servings.

SUGGESTION

Make a double recipe, keep a portion in the refrigerator to make burritos or tostados in the next few days, and freeze another portion for use in the more distant future. ❧

Dave's Rich and Zesty Burritos
❧

This is an easy dish to whip up with precooked beans (such as A Simple Pot of Beans, above.)

2 cups mashed beans
4 tortillas (Garden of Eatin' frozen whole-wheat tortillas, thawed)
½ cup chopped scallions
½ cup shredded cheddar cheese

1. In a medium-sized skillet, over low heat, sauté the mashed beans until most of the liquid has evaporated. Keep stirring as you do this so that the beans don't burn.
2. In a microwave or another frying pan heat the tortillas just until they are warm.
3. On each tortilla put a helping of beans, a sprinkling of scallions, and some cheese and roll up, tucking one end in so the filling doesn't fall out at first bite. ↜

4 servings.

Dave's Rich and Zesty Tostados
↜

Another easy, colorful, and tasty bean dish.

6 tortillas (Garden of Eatin' frozen whole-wheat tortillas, thawed)
Salt (optional)
2 cups mashed beans (A Simple Pot of Beans, page 137, or other cooked beans)
½ cup shredded cheddar cheese
1 green pepper, chopped
6 scallions, chopped
2 radishes, chopped (optional)
Pickled jalapeño pepper slices (optional)
About ½ head lettuce, shredded
1 or 2 tomatoes, chopped

1. Place tortillas, separated, on cookie sheets, sprinkle with salt if desired, and bake in a 350-degree oven until crisp. Set aside.
2. In a medium-size skillet, cook the mashed beans over low heat until most of the liquid has evaporated, stirring frequently.
3. On each crisp tortilla put a thick layer of beans and some cheddar cheese.

4. Heat in oven until cheese starts to melt.
5. Over this add some green pepper, scallions, radishes and a few slices of jalapeño if desired, shredded lettuce, and tomatoes. ✧

6 servings.

Brown Rice with Garlic
✧

The bit of oil, garlic, and chicken broth make for a tasty rice dish that can be used alone as a side dish or as the foundation for a layer of legumes. You can do this in the microwave (use a microwave-safe casserole dish) instead of on the stove in about half the time. The rice has a much different, al dente consistency prepared in a microwave compared with stove-top cooking.

1 cup brown rice
1 teaspoon olive oil
4 cloves garlic, minced (or ½ teaspoon dried garlic flakes)
2 cups chicken broth or water (if water, add salt to taste)
1 dried red chile pepper (optional)

1. Combine all ingredients in a 2-quart saucepan and bring to a boil.
2. Reduce heat to low, cover, and cook for about 45 minutes, or until all liquid is absorbed. Stir only once about halfway through for fluffy rice, and then at the end to see if all the liquid has been absorbed. ✧

4 servings.

Couscous, Chickpeas, and Vegetables
✧

This is a big recipe—it makes great leftovers. And if you are like me (I'm normally not a great lover of turnips), you won't believe how good the turnips taste in this dish.

2 cups chicken or vegetable
   bouillon, divided
1½ cups couscous
1 tablespoon oil
1 small onion, thinly sliced
Ground black pepper to taste
1 teaspoon salt
⅛ teaspoon cayenne (optional)
2 small carrots, thinly sliced
1 teaspoon cumin
¼ teaspoon cinnamon

1 small turnip, cut in matchstick
   pieces
1 small green or red bell pepper,
   diced
1 medium zucchini, quartered
   lengthwise and cut in ½-inch
   slices
15-ounce can chickpeas, drained
2 tablespoons fresh parsley,
   chopped

1. In a small saucepan bring 1½ cups of the bouillon to a boil.
2. Add the couscous, toss, cover, and set aside.
3. Heat the oil in a 6-quart kettle and sauté the onions, covered, over low heat until they are translucent.
4. Add the remaining bouillon and the pepper, salt, and cayenne, if desired.
5. Bring to a boil and add the carrots, cumin, and cinnamon.
6. Lower heat, cover, and cook for 3 minutes.
7. Add the turnip and bell pepper.
8. Cook about 5 minutes more until the turnip is tender.
9. Add the zucchini, chickpeas, and parsley and cook until the zucchini is tender.
10. Add the cooked couscous, toss to blend, correct the seasonings, and serve. ✎

10 servings.

Black-Eyed Peas and Greens
✎

Black-eyed peas and greens make for a great combination. This one has its origins in Greece, where chard is the traditional companion to the peas, but spinach works fine, too.

1½ cups black-eyed peas, soaked
   overnight in water to cover
1–1½ cups chicken bouillon
1 bay leaf
1 medium onion, chopped

2 cloves garlic, minced
1 tablespoon olive oil
1 teaspoon salt
Ground black pepper to taste
1 tablespoon fresh lemon juice

1 teaspoon fresh sage, chopped
(or ¼ teaspoon dried)

About 1 pound Swiss chard or
spinach leaves, coarsely
shredded

1. Drain the black-eyed peas and place them in a 3-quart saucepan; add the bouillon and bay leaf.
2. Bring to a boil, then lower heat and simmer, covered, until tender (about 20 minutes). Stir occasionally and add more water or bouillon as needed.
3. Meanwhile, in a small skillet, sauté the onion and garlic in the oil until translucent.
4. Add salt, pepper, lemon juice, and sage to the onion and garlic. Mix and set aside.
5. When beans are almost tender, add the greens to the saucepan and let simmer another 4–5 minutes until the greens are wilted.
6. Drain (you can reserve the excess liquid for other uses). Add the onion mixture, stir to mix, and serve.

6 servings.

Note: Use the reserved liquid to make soups or stews, or to cook some brown rice, which goes very well with this dish. ✤

Barley/Pine-Nut Casserole
✤

This is a nice alternative for rice, and works well as either a main or side dish.

1 cup pearl barley
2 tablespoons pine nuts
1 medium onion, chopped
1 tablespoon olive oil
3 cups hot chicken bouillon

¼ cup finely chopped scallions
⅓ cup finely chopped fresh
parsley
Salt and fresh-ground black
pepper to taste

1. Preheat oven to 350 degrees.
2. Rinse barley, drain, and set aside (you can do this in a colander).
3. In a small, dry skillet, toast the pine nuts, stirring, over medium heat for 3 to 5 minutes, or until lightly browned, and set aside.
4. In a 1½-quart saucepan, sauté the onion in the oil until softened.

5. Add the barley and cook, stirring constantly, for about 1 more minute, until the barley is coated with oil.
6. Stir in the stock and scallions and bring to a boil.
7. Transfer the mixture to a 1½-quart casserole dish, cover, and bake for 1 hour.
8. Remove from the oven and mix in the parsley and pine nuts.
9. Season with salt and pepper to taste. ✎

6 servings.

Barley and Vegetables
✎

This dish can be made with rice as well as barley. If you use rice, reduce the liquid to 1 cup and the salt to ¼ teaspoon.

½ cup pearl barley
1 tablespoon olive oil
1 small zucchini, chopped
4 ounces fresh mushrooms, quartered

1½ cups bouillon or broth
½ teaspoon salt, or to taste
¼ teaspoon garlic powder
¼ teaspoon ground black pepper

1. In a small, dry skillet, toast the barley over medium heat, stirring constantly, for 2–3 minutes. Transfer to a 1½-quart covered casserole.
2. Place the olive oil and zucchini in the first pan and sauté until barely tender.
3. Add the mushrooms and stir briefly.
4. Add the broth or bouillon and the seasonings, and bring to a boil.
5. Pour the mixture over the barley in the casserole and bake, covered, at 350 degrees for about 45 minutes. Check after 20 to 30 minutes and add more liquid if the casserole appears to be drying out. ✎

4 servings.

Burneta's Millet Mash

⌖

We adapted this recipe from one given to us by Burneta Clayton. We like it so much that we now make this dish with other vegetables in the cabbage family.

3 cups water
1 cup millet
1 head cauliflower, cut in chunks
2 tablespoons soy sauce
¼ teaspoon ground black pepper

½ teaspoon salt
1 teaspoon tahini (sesame-seed paste)
1 teaspoon olive oil
Dash of garlic powder

1. In a 3-quart saucepan, bring the water to a boil and add the millet, cauliflower, and soy sauce.
2. Bring to a boil again and then lower heat and cook, covered, until millet is tender.
3. Remove from heat, add all other ingredients, and mash together.
4. Pack into a small, lightly oiled casserole or loaf pan.
5. Bake in a 350-degree oven for a few minutes to reheat. ⌖

8 servings.

Black Beans and Chili Tomatoes

⌖

This is a quick, spicy meal which demonstrates how to use primarily canned ingredients with just a little extra fresh vegetables to make a dish that rivals the best you might prepare if you started everything from scratch. I've tried different canned beans and found that I prefer Progresso brand for both taste and consistency. As with many bean dishes, you can serve this over rice and top with other chopped vegetables and a sprinkle of sharp cheddar cheese.

15-ounce can Progresso black beans, with juice
10-ounce can Ro-Tel diced tomatoes and chilis
1 large carrot, sliced thin and roughly chopped
1 medium onion, chopped

Combine and mix all ingredients in a baking pan and bake, uncovered, at 350 degrees for about 45 minutes (or until the mixture reaches the consistency you prefer). The carrots and onions will still be crispy, which is the way I like them. If you want them well done, do them in the microwave for 5 minutes before blending with the beans and diced tomatoes. ✜

4 servings.

Soybean and Lima Casserole
✜

Soybeans, like tofu, are a late addition to my diet. I searched in several places for a recipe that I could recommend without reservation to others for whom soybeans might also be foreign fare, and came up with this one.

Soybeans have a much more nutty flavor and crispy consistency when ready to eat than most other legumes (they will get quite soft after many hours of cooking, but I think they lose character at that point). They are best soaked overnight before cooking, as are the limas, but the following recipe is my quick version in case you forget to do this. If you buy your soybeans in bulk, when you wash them be sure to check for any small pebbles that may still be mixed in with the beans—some pebbles look very much like beans and the packager can easily miss them. The baby lima beans take much less time to cook and are added about halfway through the entire process. I have served this recipe both as a main course and as a side dish. The basic recipe will work with just about any kind of bean or combination of beans.

1 cup soybeans	28-ounce can whole tomatoes
2 cups water (will be discarded)	6-ounce can tomato paste
2 cups chicken bouillon	1 large onion, chopped
1½ cups baby lima beans	2 teaspoons dried basil
2 cups hot water (also will be discarded)	Fresh-ground black pepper to taste

1. Wash the soybeans, place in a 3-quart saucepan with 2 cups of water, bring to a boil, remove from heat, and let sit for 2 minutes. Pour off all the water.
2. Add the chicken bouillon to the soybeans, bring to a boil, then reduce heat, cover, and simmer for 2 hours.
3. Place limas in another temporary pot or dish and cover with hot water. Let soak while the soybeans are cooking.
4. After 2 hours have passed, pour off water from lima beans and combine with the soybeans.

5. Add the whole tomatoes (with liquid), tomato paste, onion, basil, and pepper to the mixture. Stir and blend as you bring to a boil.
6. Reduce heat to low, cover, and simmer for about 2 more hours. This dish should have a thick consistency, but add liquid if necessary to your preferred level.
7. Taste toward the end of the cooking time to see if the soybeans have reached a likable consistency. Keep cooking if they are too crispy for your taste. ⊕

12 servings.

Pasta

I am very fond of pasta, as the following recipes will show. Every one of these recipes is a party dish. Once you try them you may start eating pasta several times a week. If you do, it will be much to your advantage. And don't believe that nonsense about pasta making you fat. The only way you get fat on pasta is to load it with a fatty sauce or to eat several portions at once.

Mock Lasagna
⊕

PASTA
2 cups whole-wheat elbow
    macaroni
4 cups water
1 teaspoon salt
1 tablespoon olive oil

SAUCE
1 pound low-fat ground turkey
15-ounce can tomato sauce
1 teaspoon dried basil
1 teaspoon oregano
¼ teaspoon garlic powder
¼ teaspoon chili powder
1 tablespoon dried parsley
½ teaspoon salt

FILLING
1 cup low-fat cottage cheese
8 ounces firm tofu
½ green or red bell pepper,
    chopped
6 scallions, chopped
1 tablespoon soy sauce
½ cup plain nonfat yogurt

1. Cook the macaroni in boiling salted water until al dente. Drain. Place in a bowl and toss with oil. Set aside.
2. In a nonstick pan sear the turkey until cooked with no pink remaining. Stir in the tomato sauce and spices. Bring to a boil, then lower heat and simmer for about 1 minute. Set aside.
3. Puree the cottage cheese and tofu in a food processor or blender until smooth and creamy.
4. Place in a bowl and add the bell pepper, scallions, and soy sauce. Mix.
5. Add the yogurt and mix until well blended.
6. Put half the macaroni in a 3-quart casserole. Smooth the filling over the top.
7. Cover with the rest of the macaroni and top with the sauce.
8. Bake, uncovered, in a 350-degree oven for 45 minutes. ↝

8 servings.

Nutty Pepper Pasta
↜

2 tablespoons olive oil
4 large garlic cloves, thinly sliced
½ cup coarsely chopped walnuts
2 medium bell peppers (green, red, yellow, or a combination), cored, trimmed, and cut lengthwise into ½-inch-long strips
1½ medium yellow onions, thinly sliced
10 cherry tomatoes, halved
1½ cups coarsely chopped parsley
1 teaspoon salt
Fresh-ground black pepper to taste
3 cups cooked thin spaghetti (about 6 ounces dry)
4 tablespoons grated Parmesan (optional)

1. Heat olive oil in a large skillet over medium heat.
2. Sauté garlic and walnuts till lightly browned, about 5 minutes.
3. Add the peppers and onions and cook over low heat, covered, for about 5 minutes, or until the onions are translucent.
4. Add the tomatoes and cook till soft, about 5 more minutes.

5. Add the parsley and stir to combine thoroughly. Season with salt and pepper.
6. Put the pasta in a large shallow bowl and cover with the walnut-pepper sauce.
7. Sprinkle each serving with 1 tablespoon of grated Parmesan, if desired. ⮎

4 servings.

Spaghetti with Tomatoes, Basil, and Capers
⮎

8 sun-dried tomatoes (dried, not preserved in oil)
½ pound Swiss chard, escarole, or bok choy, coarsely chopped
2 pounds tomatoes, diced
½ tablespoon capers, drained
½ cup toasted pine nuts
3 cloves garlic, minced
¼ cup grated Parmesan
4 tablespoons olive oil
½ cup fresh basil, coarsely chopped
Salt and pepper to taste
1 pound spaghetti

1. Blanch dried tomatoes in boiling water for about 2 minutes. Then remove from water and dice.
2. Wilt Swiss chard or other greens in a skillet with about 1 teaspoon of oil and a bit of water.
3. In a large bowl, combine all the ingredients except spaghetti and let them marinate.
4. Meanwhile, cook the spaghetti in boiling, salted water until it is al dente.
5. Drain, add to the tomato mixture, correct seasonings, and serve.
6. May be topped with additional Parmesan if desired.

8 servings.

Note: Combining yellow and red tomatoes makes for a very colorful dish. ⮎

Confetti Pasta with Fish and Artichokes

This is one dish that really profits from a bit of butter.

1 pound orange roughy or grouper fillets
1 tablespoon butter
1 tablespoon corn or olive oil
1 cup sliced artichoke hearts
1 each red pepper, carrot, and zucchini, cut in julienne strips
⅔ cup 1% milk and 2 teaspoons cornstarch, whisked
½ teaspoon salt
Fresh-ground pepper to taste
6 ounces angel hair pasta or vermicelli
½ cup grated Parmesan cheese
¼ teaspoon ground nutmeg

1. Cut fish in half crosswise and slice into thin strips.
2. In a 3-quart saucepan, sauté the fish in melted butter and oil; add the vegetables and cook, covered, until tender.
3. Stir in the milk/cornstarch mixture; add salt and pepper. Keep warm.
4. Cook pasta according to package directions; drain.
5. Toss well with the fish sauce and Parmesan cheese.
6. Sprinkle with nutmeg and serve immediately. ✎

6 servings.

Spinach Lasagna

This is my version of an Italian specialty that cuts the fat by two-thirds compared with the original. I like to use a combination of whole-wheat and regular lasagna noodles, mixing them up in each layer. This eliminates the mealy texture that may result when only whole-wheat noodles are used. To prevent mutilating the fresh spinach and basil use a scissors and cut to your preferred size, rather than chop. If you like a richer tomato flavor, you can use as much as 4 cups of pasta sauce to advantage in this recipe. If you use large pieces of greens your dish will pile up an inch or so above the rim of your pan, but don't worry, it shrinks down well below the rim during baking. And, in spite of my fears when I first prepared this dish, it did not drip over the sides of the pan, nor has it in the many times that have followed.

This is an excellent company dish, should you decide to serve a meat-less dinner at some special occasion, and is accompanied well by a glass of Italian red wine, such as a Bardolino. You can double the size of this recipe for a large party, in which case you should use a special lasagna pan, about 10 × 14 × 4 inches in size, and bake it 30 to 40 minutes longer. You will receive many "oohs and ahs" when you bring this large, impressive-looking dish to the table.

2 cups low-fat pasta sauce
9 lasagna noodles, soaked in very hot water for about a minute (do not cook)
12 ounces fresh mushrooms, sliced
8 ounces fresh spinach, cut into 2- to 3-inch pieces (about 4 cups)
2 ounces fresh basil, cut into 1- to 2-inch pieces (about ¾ cup, or 3 tablespoons crushed dry basil)
15 ounces part-skim ricotta cheese
8 ounces shredded part-skim mozzarella cheese
½ cup Parmesan cheese

1. Preheat oven to 350 degrees.
2. Spread some sauce over the bottom and sides of an 8×11×2-inch bak-ing dish.
3. Make three layers using, for each in order, 3 soaked lasagna noodles and one-third of the sauce, mushrooms, spinach, basil, ricotta, shred-ded mozzarella, and Parmesan.
4. Bake for about 1 hour or until browned on top.
5. Let stand for 10 minutes to let sauce settle before cutting into portions.

6 generous servings.

Note: When you double this recipe it will take longer to cook—allow at least an extra half hour. ✑

Pasta with Garlic-Clam Sauce
✑

This is a simple recipe that can be prepared quickly and served as soon as your pasta is ready. The recipe can also serve as a foundation for a vegetable-and-clam sauce. Just add a medium onion and green bell pepper, sliced, while you are sautéing the garlic, and 1 cup of sliced mushrooms when you add the clams, and you will get yet another fine vegetable/pasta treat.

8 ounces thin spaghetti
2 tablespoons olive oil
10–12 cloves garlic, minced
2 cans (about 6-ounce size) minced clams, including juice
1 small dried red chile pepper
Fresh-ground black pepper to taste
2 tablespoons grated Parmesan cheese

1. Prepare pasta according to package directions.
2. In a 3-quart saucepan, warm the oil, add the garlic, and sauté over low heat until translucent (some people like their garlic browned; it's a matter of taste and it's up to you).
3. Add the clams, chile pepper, and black pepper, and simmer while your pasta is cooking (normally about 12 minutes).
4. Add the Parmesan cheese to the sauce during the last 2 or 3 minutes of cooking.
5. While draining the pasta, pour the sauce into a serving bowl, and then add the drained pasta (less splashing than in the reverse order) and mix. (Optional: Top with another sprinkle of Parmesan cheese.) ✺

4 servings.

Once-a-Week Pasta
✺

When you look in your refrigerator crisper at the end of the week you are likely to find a few vegetables that have just passed their prime for use in a salad or in some other recipe where only the freshest can yield the flavor or texture you desire. If that happens, as it most likely will when you've been cooking a number of plant-based recipes, it's time for Once-a-Week Pasta.

Almost every vegetable, even after it's begun to grow a bit limp with age, can be added to a garlic-and-oil base for an excellent pasta sauce. Start by sautéing minced garlic in a bit of olive oil. I use 1 tablespoon of oil for every 2 servings of my final dish, and plenty of garlic, usually a whole bulb (10–12 cloves, peeled and minced). Then add, in order of the amount of time it takes to cook, whatever vegetables you find in your crisper that your intuition says might work. For example, if you have broccoli, celery, and carrots, they would go into the pot before mushrooms and spinach leaves. The tougher, more fibrous vegetables should be chopped into small pieces. As the cooking proceeds, you add ¼ to ½ cup of chicken bouillon, if necessary, to create enough sauce for the amount of pasta you plan to prepare. Don't be too quick to add this bouillon, even if the vegetables pile high and dry above your garlic and oil when you first put them in the pot. The vegetables are 80 to 95 percent water, and as they cook down, you will find your sauce expanding with healthful, tasty vegetable juices. But I frequently find the need to add a bit of bouillon, especially if I'm cooking a pound of pasta. It makes the sauce even tastier. As usual, I let each person add salt to taste when the pasta is served, at the table.

Once-a-Week Pasta is always a new and unique experience, which is what makes this dish so much fun to prepare and serve. Here is an example of a recipe that I prepared one Saturday evening with the remnants from cooking many different recipes earlier in the week. It's the kind of recipe where you just line up the things you plan to include and mince, chop, or slice one item at a time and add it to the sauce as you go along. Since the sauce can simmer for quite a time to advantage, I usually wait to start my pasta until I'm near the end of my preparations for the sauce.

¼ cup olive oil
12 cloves garlic, minced
4 stalks broccoli, about an inch of the toughest, lower stalk removed, and the rest chopped in small pieces
2 leeks, sliced thin
¼ white onion, chopped
2 stalks celery, chopped
1 large green bell pepper, diced
½ large red bell pepper, diced
1 small piece napa cabbage (the heart), chopped
3 large mushrooms, sliced
1 ounce fresh spinach
¼ to ½ cup chicken bouillon (optional)
3 or 4 dried hot red peppers (optional, but strongly recommended)
Fresh-ground black pepper to taste
4 tablespoons shredded or grated Parmesan
1 pound favorite pasta, cooked

1. Warm the oil in a 3-quart or larger saucepan, add the minced garlic, and sauté over low heat until translucent.

2. Add the chopped broccoli to the garlic and oil, cover, and begin simmering over low heat.
3. Prepare, one at a time (my projected order of required cooking time), leeks, onion, celery, green and red bell pepper, napa cabbage, mushrooms, and spinach. Add to the sauce, stir, cover the pot, and simmer in between additions. (Toward the end of these preparations, I put the water on to heat for my pasta, which should be cooked al dente.)
4. If the sauce does not appear to have enough liquid, add the bouillon.
5. Add the dried hot red peppers (optional), black pepper, and Parmesan cheese and stir. Continue simmering until pasta is done.
6. Drain the pasta, pour the sauce into a spacious casserole dish, and add the pasta to the sauce. Mix and top with some extra Parmesan if desired. If necessary, place in a warm oven (under 200 degrees) until serving time.

8 generous servings.

I have also used carrots, zucchini, yellow summer squash, tomatoes, cucumbers, various greens and cabbages (including cauliflower and turnips), garbanzos, lettuce, and herbs such as parsley and basil in my Once-a-Week Pasta sauce. ❧

Tofu

My wife, Enid, who was in charge of our venture into the world of tofu cookery, sent me this little note with these recipes after she had finished editing them and checking for errors:

"Tofu? You gotta be kidding!" That was my initial reaction to even thinking about working with tofu. But I've changed completely on that subject. The dishes that follow are among my favorites. The recipes all use firm tofu (there are other kinds) because that seemed to be the easiest to work with, and it's now available in most supermarkets as well as health-food stores. If you don't have much experience preparing tofu, the simplest recipe to start, and with which to win acceptance from family and friends if they haven't already been introduced to tofu, is the Scalloped Potatoes and Tofu. Next I'd suggest Curried Tofu and Cabbage. While I liked these dishes myself, I was amazed at how much our friends and tasters liked them. Tofu is a very versatile food—I have even modified my favorite chocolate cheesecake recipe, substituting tofu for one of the cheeses (page 180). The flavor and consistency are even closer to the original, super-high-fat version than ever. I hope you will enjoy these recipes, and remember, if you don't use the entire package of tofu in a recipe, the remainder keeps very well for up to a week if you put it in a container and cover with cold water. Change the water every day until you use it all up. For much useful information about tofu and many good recipes, I recommend *Tofu Cookery* by Louise Hagler (Summertown, Tenn.: The Book Publishing Company, 1982). Several of my own recipes are based on hers, modified to our tastes.

Scalloped Potatoes and Tofu
✧

1 tablespoon butter
2 tablespoons whole-wheat flour
1⅓ cups 1% milk
½ teaspoon salt
Fresh-ground pepper to taste
¼ teaspoon garlic powder
¼ teaspoon caraway seeds
½ cup pitted sliced black olives

2 medium potatoes, thinly sliced
¼ pound firm tofu, drained and
   thinly sliced
4 tablespoons shredded cheddar
4 tablespoons stuffing mix or
   breadcrumbs

1. Melt butter in medium saucepan.
2. Add the flour and stir until all the flour is moistened.
3. Add the milk and cook, stirring, over low heat, until the mixture thickens.
4. Add the seasonings, caraway seeds, and olives. Mix well and set aside.
5. In an oiled casserole dish, place half the potatoes topped with half the tofu.
6. Cover with half the sauce.
7. Repeat.
8. Cover and bake in a 350-degree oven for 45 minutes.
9. Uncover and sprinkle with cheese and stuffing mix or breadcrumbs.
10. Return to oven and bake 15 minutes longer or until potatoes are tender. ✧

6 servings.

Potato-Tofu Casserole

~

3 cups cooked potatoes, mashed
1½ pounds firm tofu, mashed
1 teaspoon salt
¼ teaspoon black pepper
½ teaspoon garlic powder
¼ cup fresh parsley, chopped

2 teaspoons fresh chives, snipped
   small
1 medium onion, chopped
2 tablespoons olive oil
Paprika

1. Preheat oven to 325 degrees.
2. In a medium-size bowl mix together the potatoes, tofu, salt, pepper, garlic powder, parsley, and chives.
3. In a small skillet, sauté onion in the oil.
4. When the onions are soft and translucent, stir into the potato-tofu mixture.
5. Spread into an oiled 8×8×2-inch baking dish, and sprinkle with paprika.
6. Bake for 35 minutes. ~

6 servings.

Curried Tofu and Cabbage

~

¼ cup soy sauce
½ teaspoon cumin
½ teaspoon cardamom
½ teaspoon cinnamon
½ teaspoon turmeric
1 teaspoon salt
1 clove garlic, crushed
½ pound firm tofu, cut into small
   cubes

1 tablespoon olive oil
1 small cabbage, cored and sliced
2 cups chopped celery
1 small onion, chopped
1 sprig fresh parsley, chopped
1 teaspoon grated or minced
   fresh ginger (or 1 teaspoon
   ground ginger)

1. Place the soy sauce and the next 6 ingredients in a small bowl. Add the cubed tofu and let it marinate while you prepare the rest of the vegetables.
2. With a slotted spoon, remove the tofu from the marinade and sauté in the oil in a large skillet until slightly browned.

3. Add the remaining ingredients and cook, covered, for 5–10 minutes over medium-low heat until the vegetables are as tender as you like them, stirring frequently. ❧

6 servings.

Broccoli Walnut Stir-Fry
❧

This dish is served hot over brown or wild rice.

1 cup water
½ teaspoon salt
2 carrots, thinly sliced
1 bunch broccoli (use just the flowerets, and 1 inch of the stem, reserving the remainder of the stalks for pasta sauce or soups)
1 pound firm tofu, cut in 1-inch cubes
2 tablespoons oil (divided)
2 onions, thinly sliced
1 cup mushrooms, sliced
1 cup walnuts
1 tablespoon cornstarch
3 tablespoons tamari sauce (or regular soy sauce)
¼ teaspoon crushed hot red pepper

1. Using a 2-quart saucepan, bring water and salt to a boil and drop in the carrots and broccoli. Cook 1 minute then drain, reserving the liquid.
2. In a large skillet, brown the tofu lightly in 1 tablespoon of the oil over medium heat.
3. With a slotted spoon, remove from skillet and reserve.
4. Put the remainder of the oil in the skillet and sauté the onions over medium heat.
5. Add the mushrooms, walnuts, carrots, and broccoli and stir.
6. Add the tofu and stir.
7. To the reserved vegetable liquid add the cornstarch, tamari sauce, and hot red pepper. Pour over the vegetables and tofu, stir, and cook until bubbling. ❧

4 servings.

Spiced Tofu Loaf

This savory loaf is excellent cold the next day in sandwiches.

1½ pounds firm tofu, mashed	¼ teaspoon ground ginger
½ cup tomato sauce	½ teaspoon dried basil
2 tablespoons soy sauce	½ teaspoon dried thyme
1 tablespoon Dijon mustard	1 medium onion, chopped
¼ cup Egg Beaters	1 clove garlic, crushed
½ cup chopped fresh parsley	1 cup stuffing mix
¼ teaspoon ground black pepper	1 tablespoon olive oil

1. Preheat oven to 350 degrees.
2. Mix together all ingredients, except oil.
3. Use the oil to lightly cover the bottom and sides of a loaf pan.
4. Press the mixture into the pan and bake the loaf for about 1 hour.
5. Let cool for 10–15 minutes before removing from the pan.
6. Slice and serve in the manner of a meat loaf. ✧

8 servings.

Textured Vegetable Protein

A short time after discovering the many uses of tofu, we began experimenting with textured (also called texturized) vegetable protein. While textured vegetable protein can be made from grain such as wheat, we use defatted soy flour in our own preparations. The acronym "TVP" is commonly used to mean any kind of textured vegetable protein, but it is actually a registered trademark of the Archer Daniels Midland Company, so when you see a product labeled TVP®, that product will have been produced from soy flour and not some other grain.

We obtain generic defatted soy flour (it does not carry the TVP trademark) in bulk from our health-food store where it comes in various forms, including granules, flakes, and chunks. If only the chunks are available in your area, they can be ground down to granule size in a food processor.

Textured vegetable protein from soy flour is fat free and, like tofu, is quite tasteless and takes on the flavor of herbs and spices. It has much more body than tofu, and meat-loaf analogues can be made with different textures from very firm to soft, depending upon how much flour or breadcrumbs you add, as I indicate in my recipe for Meatless Meat Loaf.

If you are looking for vegetable dishes that resemble meat dishes in taste and texture, I recommend you try the two recipes that follow. They are my versions of recipes in *The TVP® Cookbook* by Dorothy R. Bates (Summertown, Tenn.: The Book Publishing Company, 1991).

Meatless Meat Loaf

The high-gluten whole-wheat flour that we buy in our health-food store and use in this recipe gives our loaf a very firm texture. If you like a softer texture, use a fifty-fifty mixture of breadcrumbs and flour.

3 cups textured soy protein granules
2¼ cups boiling water
8 ounces tomato sauce
1 medium onion, chopped
1 tablespoon olive oil
¾ cup high-gluten whole-wheat flour (or 50/50 flour and breadcrumbs)
2 tablespoons tamari sauce
1 tablespoon Worcestershire sauce
¼ teaspoon fresh-ground black pepper
1 teaspoon each garlic powder, basil, oregano, and marjoram
½ cup fresh parsley, minced

1. Place the soy granules in a large mixing bowl, add the boiling water and tomato sauce, mix well, and let stand for 10 minutes.
2. Place the chopped onion and oil in a microwave-safe dish and microwave until soft (about 3 minutes) or sauté until soft on the stove in a small skillet.
3. Add onions and all remaining ingredients to the rehydrated soy granules and mix well.
4. Put the mixture in a lightly oiled loaf or bread pan, 9 × 5 × 2½ inches (or a suitably sized casserole), and press down firmly with a large spoon, smoothing the top.
5. Bake at 350 degrees for 45 minutes, or until firm (if it begins to brown too deeply before it is done, cover with aluminum foil).
6. Remove from oven, let stand for 10 minutes, run a knife around the edges, and turn loaf out on a platter.

8 servings.

This loaf goes well with Onion Gravy (page 173), and it's excellent the next day in sandwiches. I sometimes make a spicy version in a large casserole, covered with tomato sauce (a 16-ounce can) and sprinkled with cayenne pepper before baking. ⌒

Creole Stew
⌒

This dish goes well with a starch, for example, over rice, a baked potato, or pasta.

1 cup textured soy protein chunks	16-ounce can stewed tomatoes
1 tablespoon ketchup	3 cloves garlic, minced
1 cup boiling water	½ teaspoon salt
1 tablespoon olive oil	½ teaspoon cumin powder
1 medium onion, chopped	1 bay leaf
1 green bell pepper, chopped	Cayenne pepper to taste

1. In a microwave-safe dish, combine the soy chunks, ketchup, and boiling water. Let it stand for 10 minutes and then microwave on medium high for 10 minutes. (If you don't have a microwave combine the ingredients in a suitable stove-top pan and simmer for 20 minutes.)
2. Combine the olive oil, onion, and pepper in a large skillet and sauté until soft (about 3 to 5 minutes).
3. Add the tomatoes and the remaining ingredients to the onions and simmer over low heat for 20 minutes.
4. Add the cooked soy chunks to the sauce and cook for 5 minutes.
5. Remove the bay leaf before serving. ⌒

6 servings.

Vegetables

I have heard a number of reasons why people don't make plant foods, in particular vegetables, a main part of their diets. First is a simple "I don't like them," which is closely followed by "Too much bother" or, by the cook in the family, "My family won't eat them." If any of these reasons apply to you, I hope my recipes will change all that. Vegetables are really easy to prepare and a snap to season in tempting ways. Before going on to the more complex or unusual recipes in this section, here are hints for some simple and quick ways to prepare a number of different kinds of vegetables.

Greens can be microwaved, steamed, or simmered in a little water for several minutes, drained, and seasoned with Herb Salt, Traditional Italian Herb Blend, or one of the garam masalas (pages 181–83). It takes just a bit of oil (I use olive oil, about 1 teaspoon for 10 ounces of spinach and the like) to give greens a more pleasant feeling in the mouth, and bring out the flavors of the other seasonings. My favorite way to make fresh greens is to sauté them in olive oil with a few cloves of garlic (minced). Start the garlic in a large skillet with about 1 tablespoon of oil. Cook until translucent, then add a pile of greens (all the pan will hold) and sauté only until wilted. Delicious!

Winter squash of all varieties can be split in half, and baked face-down on a shallow, foil-lined baking pan. I put a little oil, salt, and pepper on the foil, and swish the squash around in it before placing in the oven. It takes about 45 minutes at 350 degrees for the average-sized acorn or butternut squash. Turn open side up for the last 10 minutes of baking to get rid of excess moisture in the vegetable. If you like your squash on the sweet side, you can sprinkle on other seasonings, such as cinnamon and brown sugar, just before the final 10 minutes of baking.

Beets can be baked like potatoes; cut off the tops and roots, leaving about an inch of each attached, wrap in foil, and bake for about 45 minutes at 350 degrees. Remove from the foil and peel off the top layer of skin. Cut up and season with a little oil, salt, and pepper.

Non-leafy vegetables such as *celery, carrots, and summer squash* can all be microwaved, steamed, or baked (with added liquid). My preferred method is in the microwave. It's convenient, quick, and is said to preserve the most nutritional value. For example, carrots and celery, sliced thin, take 7 to 10 minutes in the microwave, and can be quickly seasoned with a teaspoon of oil, a bit of salt and pepper, and a bit of honey (half a teaspoon for a recipe containing 2 large carrots and 2 large stalks of celery). With summer squash I use a conventional oven: just thinly slice the squash, place in a large casserole, cover with a can of whole tomatoes (cut these into smaller pieces after adding to the casserole), sprinkle with Parmesan cheese, breadcrumbs, and other seasonings (such as garlic and onion powder), and bake, uncovered, for 30 to 45 minutes at 350 degrees.

The seasonings and general approaches used in many of the recipes that follow can be applied to a number of other vegetables—just use your imagination and follow your instincts or preferences.

Here are some suggestions on selecting and storing fruits and vegetables to conserve their cancer-fighting nutrients:

- Avoid damaged or wilted produce since rough handling and aging can increase loss of vitamins.
- Find out when your supermarket receives its produce and shop on those days. Eat the vegetables soon thereafter since vitamin content and flavor begin to deteriorate after 4 or 5 days.
- Fresh and frozen produce tend to retain more nourishment than canned.
- Allow fresh fruit and vegetables to ripen, then refrigerate immediately. This helps to preserve vitamins A, C, and folate, and other nutrients.
- Do not wash produce before storing since washing increases the rate of deterioration. Wash produce just before using. This also preserves water-soluble vitamins B and C, and other nutrients.
- Frozen vegetables as well as other frozen foods should be kept at 0 degrees Fahrenheit or lower to preserve nutrients and prevent spoilage.
- When cutting up produce for use, remember that large chunks have less area exposed to air and lose nutrients more slowly than small chunks.
- Thoroughly wash all produce before using to remove pesticide residues. Although it's deemed safe, I believe you should choose produce with the least amount of waxy preservative. Locally grown fruit (such as apples) and vegetables (such as cucumbers) will usually have less of a preservative coating than those brought from afar, which require longer periods of storage.
- To avoid pesticides and preservatives as much as possible, choose organically grown produce, but you should be aware that plants produce their own natural pesticides to ward off insects and these can be as toxic to humans as artificial pesticides. Your best guarantee of avoiding too great a concentration of any toxic compound and of obtaining the greatest variety of nutrients and chemopreventive phytochemicals is to eat a wide variety of different fruits and vegetables, obtained from different plots of ground, and not too much of the same food every day.

About the numbers of servings suggested for these recipes: The numbers are for very generous serving sizes, often 50 percent or more larger than the ½ cup considered to be a serving in the USDA guidelines for cooked vegetables. That's because I expect you to ultimately be combining 2, 3, or even more vegetable dishes for meatless main meals. If you are keeping track of servings, take this into consideration. For example, if you serve a full cup of Roasted Vegetables with a large baked potato or a cup of rice, that's 2 vegetable servings and 2 grain servings according to USDA portion guidelines.

Asparagus and Pine Nuts

How do you cook asparagus so that the tender tips get done at the same time as the tougher stems? My preferred way is in a special asparagus cooker, in the microwave. The special asparagus cooker holds the asparagus upright. You place enough water in the cooker to cover just the stems. Then microwave according to your oven's directions (usually 7 to 10 minutes on high). The tips, cooking in the steam, will not turn to mush when the stems are done cooking in the water.

2 bunches asparagus, cooked
   until just tender
2 tablespoons pine nuts
2 teaspoons butter

4 teaspoons water
2 cloves garlic, crushed
Salt and pepper to taste

1. Toast the pine nuts in a nonstick pan, stirring constantly, until they are golden brown. Remove and place in a small bowl.
2. Melt the butter in the water in the same pan.
3. Add the garlic, salt, and pepper and cook until the garlic starts to brown.
4. Add the garlic mixture to the pine nuts and then sprinkle over the cooked asparagus. Toss gently and serve.

4 servings.

Herbed Potatoes

Each herb in this recipe adds a distinctive flavor. You can use the oil, lemon juice, and herb mixture on a plain baked potato when you don't wish to slice up the potatoes first. It will taste a little different for not having gone through the baking process, but still very good.

4 medium potatoes, thinly sliced
2 tablespoons + 1 teaspoon corn
   oil (divided)
2 tablespoons lemon juice
1 teaspoon salt

½ teaspoon each rosemary, sage,
   and thyme
¼ teaspoon each garlic powder,
   onion powder, and pepper

1. Grease a casserole dish with a teaspoon of oil.
2. Combine all other ingredients, place in the casserole, and bake, covered, for 30 minutes at 350 degrees. Uncover and cook 20 to 30 minutes more (longer for crisper potatoes). ❧

6 servings.

Roasted Rosemary Potatoes
❧

With red potatoes this is an especially pretty dish.

8 small red potatoes (or 2 large Idahos)
1 tablespoon fresh rosemary, chopped (or 1 teaspoon dried, crushed)
1 tablespoon olive oil
1 tablespoon lemon juice
1 teaspoon salt
Ground black pepper to taste
½ teaspoon garlic powder
⅛ teaspoon crushed red pepper (optional)

1. Preheat oven to 350 degrees.
2. Cut the potatoes into small chunks.
3. Combine all other ingredients and pour over the potatoes, tossing to coat evenly.
4. Place on a baking sheet and roast for 30–45 minutes or until tender, turning now and then. ❧

4 servings.

Curried Chickpeas and Potatoes
❧

The Indian-style spice mixture in this dish (turmeric, fennel seed, coriander, ginger, and crushed red pepper) is called a garam masala or curry (see page 181 for other garam masalas). When you find ones you like, you can use them to season a variety of vegetables and legumes.

1 tablespoon olive oil
2 garlic cloves, minced
1 medium onion, chopped
6–8 green onions, including 3 inches of their green stems, cut in 1-inch pieces

1 tablespoon turmeric
1 teaspoon ground coriander
½ teaspoon fennel seed, crushed with mortar and pestle
¼ teaspoon crushed red pepper
1 teaspoon ginger
1 cup V8 juice
1 cup vegetable or chicken broth
3 medium potatoes, cut in 1-inch chunks
15-ounce can chickpeas, drained and rinsed
½ teaspoon minced jalapeño pepper (optional)
1 teaspoon salt

1. Heat the oil in a medium saucepan.
2. Add the garlic and both types of onions; sauté until the vegetables are soft.
3. Stir in the spices and sauté for 30 seconds.
4. Add the remaining ingredients, cover, and simmer for about 40 minutes, or until the potatoes are tender. ᴥ

4 servings.

Cauliflower du Barry

(Potatoes and Cauliflower)
ᴥ

Different recipes for this dish vary the relative amounts of cauliflower and potatoes. One calls for 4 parts cauliflower to 1 part potatoes, and recommends that they be mashed together with cream and eaten with fried bread. I like a bit more potatoes, and prefer to skip the cream and fried bread.

2 large potatoes, cut into small chunks
1 small head cauliflower, flowerets and 1 inch of stem only
1½ cups water

1 tablespoon butter
½ teaspoon nutmeg
Ground black pepper to taste
1–1½ teaspoons salt
¼ teaspoon garlic powder

1. Cook the potatoes and cauliflower together in the water (to cover) until tender.
2. Drain, reserving liquid.

3. Mash. Mix in the butter and spices.
4. Add some of the cauliflower/potato water if more liquid is needed. ⊕

8 servings.

Dusty Cauliflower

This is a favorite appetizer, with great eye appeal, and it works very well
as a side dish. You can prepare mushrooms the same way. We have sometimes made both mushrooms and cauliflower for dinner parties.

4 cups cauliflower flowerets	4 teaspoons grated Parmesan
2 tablespoons oil	⅛ teaspoon ground black pepper
3 tablespoons oat bran	Dash garlic powder
3 tablespoons breadcrumbs	¼ teaspoon salt

1. Preheat oven to 400 degrees.
2. Lightly oil a shallow baking pan.
3. Combine cauliflower and oil in a large mixing bowl and toss to coat.
4. Combine all other ingredients in another bowl, then pour over the cauliflower and toss to coat.
5. Spread in the prepared pan and bake for 18–20 minutes until lightly
   browned. ⊕

4 servings.

Broccoflower Puree

People who don't like the texture of cauliflower or broccoli find that a
puree, with seasonings such as these, makes for an attractive dish.

1 small onion, chopped	¼ teaspoon salt
1 clove garlic, minced	1 head broccoflower (or
1 teaspoon sesame or other oil	cauliflower), cut into flowerets
1 tablespoon + ¼ cup water	1 tablespoon soy sauce
(divided)	Pepper to taste

1. Cook the onion and garlic with the oil and 1 tablespoon of water in a microwave, covered, on high for about 3 minutes or until onion is translucent.
2. Add salt, broccoflower, and ¼ cup of water.
3. Cook on high for 8–10 minutes until tender.
4. Place all in a food processor or blender with the soy sauce and pepper.
5. Blend and serve. ⊷

4 servings.

Brussels Sprouts with Garlic and Oil
⊷

I have yet to meet a person who did not like brussels sprouts prepared according to this and the following recipe.

1 pound fresh brussels sprouts (remove outer leaves, and cut in half
   if very large), steamed or microwaved until tender
2 or more cloves garlic, minced
2 teaspoons olive oil
1 or 2 tablespoons breadcrumbs

1. In a skillet large enough to hold the sprouts, begin by sautéing the garlic in oil on low heat until either translucent or lightly browned (browning it gives it a stronger, slightly bitter flavor).
2. Add cooked brussels sprouts and breadcrumbs, and continue on low heat until the breadcrumbs are crisp (about 15 minutes).
3. Serve, letting each individual add salt and/or pepper, if desired, at the table. ⊷

4 servings.

Parmesan-Dill Brussels Sprouts
⊷

1 pound fresh brussels sprouts
¼ cup water
½ teaspoon salt
1 tablespoon fresh lemon juice
1 tablespoon grated Parmesan

2 teaspoons olive oil (or butter, melted)
½ teaspoon dried dill weed
Ground black pepper to taste

1. Wash sprouts and remove tough outer leaves. Make a shallow cut in the bottoms of the stems. If some of the sprouts are very large you may want to halve them.
2. Microwave, covered lightly, with the water and salt for 7–9 minutes on high, mixing after 4 minutes. Check for tenderness and, if done, drain, place in serving dish, and toss with other ingredients. ✺

4 servings.

Creamy Cabbage
✺

This is a good side dish with a fish, chicken, or starchy main course.

½ large cabbage, coarsely
   chopped
¼ cup water
¼ teaspoon salt
1 tablespoon butter
1 tablespoon cabbage water
2 tablespoons whole-wheat flour

1 cup 1% milk
1 tablespoon nutritional yeast
⅛ teaspoon cayenne
   ¼ teaspoon tarragon
¼ teaspoon salt
3 tablespoons breadcrumbs or
   stuffing mix

1. Microwave chopped cabbage with ¼ cup water and ¼ teaspoon salt for about 9 minutes on high, stirring once after 5 minutes.
2. Drain, reserving cabbage water, and place in lightly oiled casserole dish.
3. Melt butter in a small saucepan with 1 tablespoon of the cabbage water.
4. Add the flour and stir until moistened.
5. Add the milk and whisk or stir over low heat until the flour dissolves.
6. Add yeast, spices, and salt. Continue cooking and stirring until the sauce begins to thicken.
7. Pour the sauce over the cabbage and sprinkle with breadcrumbs or stuffing mix.
8. Bake at 350 degrees for about 30 minutes or until bubbly. ✺

6 servings.

Bok Choy and Mushrooms

The soy sauce and A-1 steak sauce yield a seasoning similar to an Oriental oyster sauce (I have never found a commercial version that I liked). This dish can be served over brown rice.

¼ pound mushrooms, quartered
1 tablespoon olive oil
½ pound bok choy (or other green, leafy cabbage), coarsely chopped
4 teaspoons soy sauce
1 teaspoon A-1 steak sauce

1. Stir-fry mushrooms in heated oil for about 2 minutes.
2. Add bok choy and stir-fry 1–2 minutes, until wilted.
3. Add soy sauce and steak sauce and simmer, partially covered, for 2–3 minutes more. ⊕

4 servings.

Rosemary Carrots

3 cups thinly sliced carrots
1 teaspoon bouillon granules
¼ cup water
1 teaspoon brown sugar
1 teaspoon oil

¼ teaspoon dried rosemary, crushed
1 teaspoon dried chives
⅛ teaspoon pepper

1. Put the carrots in a microwave-safe casserole dish.
2. Combine the other ingredients and pour over the carrots.
3. Cover and microwave on high for 6–9 minutes until carrots are tender, stirring once after 5 minutes. ⊕

6 servings.

Carrots and Celery

5 carrots, sliced thin
5 stalks celery, sliced thin
¼ cup water
¼ teaspoon salt
Ground pepper to taste

1½ teaspoons olive oil
1½ teaspoons fresh chopped
   chives
1½ teaspoons vegetable water

1. Combine the first 4 ingredients in a microwave-safe bowl, cover, and microwave for about 15 minutes, stirring after 7 minutes.
2. Drain, reserving 1½ teaspoons of the vegetable liquid, and put carrots and celery in a serving bowl.
3. Heat, covered, the remaining 4 ingredients in the original microwave bowl until warm (about 30 seconds on high), pour over carrots and celery, and toss.
4. Add more salt and pepper if necessary.

6 servings.

Fresh Beets

1 bunch fresh beets (about 1¼
   pounds without leaves)
½ cup water
½ teaspoon salt

1 small onion, chopped
1½ teaspoons olive oil
1 teaspoon butter
Pepper to taste

1. Remove stems of beets to about 1 inch from beet.
2. Trim tails the same.
3. Wash well under running water.
4. Place in microwave-safe casserole dish with water and salt.
5. Cover and microwave for 22–25 minutes, stirring after 11 minutes.
6. When the beets are tender and cool enough to handle, peel them and cut into small chunks.
7. Put into a small casserole and keep warm.
8. In a small skillet, sauté the onion in the oil and butter over low heat until tender.
9. Pour over beets, add pepper to taste, toss lightly, and serve.

3 servings.

Roasted Vegetables

A feast for the eyes as well as the palate. A large serving of this dish with a starchy vegetable can make a complete meal.

2 leeks, cut into 1-inch slices
4 small yellow squash, cut in 1-inch slices
4 zucchini, cut in 1-inch slices
2 large red or yellow onions, cut in eighths
2 tablespoons olive oil
2 teaspoons dried oregano
1 teaspoon salt
½ teaspoon ground black pepper
½ teaspoon garlic powder
2 large red bell peppers, cut in ½-inch strips
2 large yellow bell peppers, cut in ½-inch strips
1 tablespoon lemon juice
¼ cup chopped parsley

1. Preheat oven to 500 degrees.
2. Toss the first 4 ingredients with the olive oil and seasonings.
3. Spread in a large baking pan and bake for 10 minutes.
4. Add peppers and toss gently.
5. Spread out and bake for 10 minutes more or until vegetables are tender and show just a bit of charring.
6. Place in a bowl, let cool a bit, and then toss gently with the lemon juice and parsley. ↩

6 servings.

Tri-Color Pepper Sauté

This beautiful recipe tastes as good as it looks. You can make it with just one kind of bell pepper if you like, but the three colors make it especially attractive.

6 medium bell peppers, 2 each red, yellow, and green
2 tablespoons olive oil
1 teaspoon red wine vinegar
½ teaspoon sugar
⅓ cup drained capers
4 tablespoons drained, chopped pimiento-stuffed olives
2 teaspoons dried oregano, crushed

1. Remove stems and seeds from peppers and cut into quarters.
2. Sauté, covered, in the oil until softened.
3. Mix in the remaining ingredients.
4. Simmer, covered, for about 20 minutes, or until peppers are tender, but not mushy. ❧

6 servings.

Mediterranean-Style Spinach
❧

This method of preparation can be used with just about any variety of greens, fresh or frozen.

2 cloves garlic, crushed
1 tablespoon olive oil
2 10-ounce packages frozen chopped spinach, defrosted and drained well
Salt and ground pepper to taste
2 tablespoons feta cheese

1. In a 2-quart saucepan sauté the garlic in the olive oil until translucent.
2. Add spinach, salt, and pepper, mix, and cook, covered, for about 5–7 minutes.
3. Add feta cheese and toss to blend. ❧

4 servings.

Spinach Casserole
❧

6 tablespoons whole-wheat flour
½ teaspoon each onion powder and garlic powder
1 teaspoon each salt and dry mustard
Dash of cayenne (optional)
1 tablespoon each fresh chopped chives, sage, and tarragon (if fresh herbs are unavailable, use 1 teaspoon each dried)
½ cup Egg Beaters (equivalent to 2 eggs)
2 10-ounce packages frozen spinach, defrosted and drained (save juice for soup)
½ cup shredded cheddar cheese

1 cup plain, fat-free yogurt
3 tablespoons breadcrumbs or stuffing mix

1. In a large bowl, combine wheat flour, spices, herbs, and Egg Beaters, and beat until smooth.
2. Add spinach, cheese, and yogurt and blend.
3. Put into a lightly oiled casserole dish, top with breadcrumbs or stuffing mix, and bake for about 45 minutes at 350 degrees. ✺

4 servings.

Green-Bean Ragout

(Fassolakia Yiahni)
✺

This dish can be eaten hot or cold with equal enjoyment, and it can be made with just about any variety of snap bean.

2 tablespoons olive oil
2 tablespoons water
2 onions, chopped
1½ pounds fresh green beans, tops and tails removed
3 medium potatoes, peeled and quartered
2 garlic cloves, crushed

4 ripe tomatoes, coarsely chopped
¼ cup water
Salt and fresh-ground black pepper to taste
1 teaspoon dried basil
6 tablespoons feta cheese, crumbled

1. Heat the oil and 2 tablespoons of water in a large saucepan and add the onions. Cook on medium-low for 3–4 minutes, or until softened but not browned.
2. Add the green beans and the potatoes and stir to coat with oil.
3. Add the garlic and cook for another 5 minutes.
4. Add the tomatoes and the ¼ cup of water.
5. Add salt, pepper, and basil, reduce the heat, and simmer, covered, for about 1½ hours, or until the beans and potatoes are soft, adding a little extra water if necessary.
6. Sprinkle with the crumbled feta cheese. ✺

6 servings.

Green-Bean Casserole

⌒

3 10-ounce packages frozen
    french-cut green beans
1 medium onion, chopped
1 clove garlic, crushed
2 teaspoons butter and 4
    teaspoons water
4 tablespoons whole-wheat flour
1 cup 1% milk
½ cup plain nonfat yogurt

4 tablespoons Parmesan cheese,
    grated or shredded
1 tablespoon nutritional yeast
1 teaspoon salt
¼ teaspoon ground black pepper
Dash of cayenne (optional)
3 tablespoons stuffing mix or
    breadcrumbs

1. Preheat oven to 350 degrees.
2. Cook the green beans according to the package directions and drain
   (you can freeze the liquid for later use in soup). Put them in a medium-
   sized bowl and set aside.
3. In a small skillet, sauté onion and garlic in the butter/water mixture until
   tender.
4. Sprinkle the flour over the onion mixture and blend until the flour is
   moistened.
5. Add the milk and cook until thickened.
6. Add this mixture to the beans.
7. Combine all other ingredients, except the stuffing mix, with the beans.
8. Place the beans in a greased casserole dish, sprinkle the stuffing mix
   on top, and bake for 20–25 minutes. ⌒

6 servings.

Zucchini Boats

⌒

1 small zucchini per person
Boiling water
Olive oil
Garlic powder

¼ teaspoon grated Parmesan per
    half zucchini
Pepper and salt

1. In a kettle large enough to hold all the whole zucchinis you intend to
   cook, bring about 1 inch of water to a boil.

2. Put the whole zucchinis in and lower the heat. Cook about 5 minutes.
3. Remove the zucchinis with a slotted spoon and let cool.
4. When cool enough to handle, cut each in half lengthwise.
5. Score the tops with a fork, brush with oil, and sprinkle with garlic powder, Parmesan, pepper, and salt.
6. Bake at 350 degrees for about 10 minutes. ✌

Serving size is 1 zucchini per person (2 halves).

Gravy and Sauce

Here are a simple, tasty gravy and a meat sauce (made with turkey) for pasta or rice.

Onion Gravy
✌

This recipe is based on one by Burneta Clayton and is good over her Millet Mash (page 143) and other similar dishes.

1 teaspoon sesame oil
2 teaspoons water
1 onion, chopped
1/8 teaspoon garlic powder
1/4 teaspoon ground ginger

1/4 teaspoon salt
1 tablespoon soy sauce
1 cup water (divided)
1 tablespoon cornstarch

1. In a small saucepan combine the oil and 2 teaspoons of water.
2. Add the onion and sauté, partially covered, over medium heat, stirring often, until onions are translucent and are just barely starting to brown.
3. Add the spices and soy sauce.
4. Add water, reserving 2 tablespoons.
5. Cook, covered, until the onions are tender.
6. Combine the cornstarch with the reserved water and blend.
7. Add to the onions and cook until the gravy thickens. ✌

About 1½ cups gravy; serving size is ¼ cup.

Dave's Hearty Meat Sauce

1 pound lean ground turkey
1 medium onion, chopped
3 cloves garlic, minced
1 green or red bell pepper,
  chopped
15-ounce can tomato sauce
15-ounce can whole tomatoes

6-ounce (drained weight) can
  medium pitted black olives,
  drained and rinsed
1 cup V8 or other vegetable
  juice
½ teaspoon salt
1 teaspoon basil
1 teaspoon oregano
⅛ teaspoon cayenne

1. In a large skillet brown the turkey until no pink remains.
2. Lift out with a slotted spoon and reserve.
3. Braise onion, garlic, and bell pepper, covered, in the same pan. If there is no juice left from the turkey, add a little water.
4. When onions are translucent, add canned goods, turkey, and vegetable juice.
5. Add spices.
6. Bring to a boil, cover, lower heat, and simmer for about 2 hours, stirring occasionally. ↽

8 servings.

Desserts

A treat need not be a "cheat" when you use wholesome ingredients. We often use whole-wheat flour in place of unbleached white flour, but if the product seems too heavy for you, try whole-wheat pastry flour (it's had a small bit of the fibrous portion removed) or mix whole-wheat flour with unbleached white flour. Most of our recipes are half-fat versions of traditional recipes, with skim or 1% milk, Egg Beaters, nonfat yogurt, and low-fat sour cream replacing the higher-fat original ingredients. You can usually do the same with any of your favorite recipes, but it may take a little experimentation.

However, we still prefer butter to margarine or oil as the fat in many recipes—sometimes nothing can replace butter for flavor and texture. But it's minimal, and as long as you stick with 1 serving you won't be adding but a gram or two of saturated fat to your diet. Please remember that you cannot eat 2 or 3 portions of a nonfat or low-fat version of a food in place of a single portion of the high-fat food and come out ahead of the game. You will end up with more calories, if not more fat.

My wife, Enid, is especially fond of chocolate and has worked very hard to come up with healthier, lower-fat versions of her favorites: a Chewy Cocoa Cake with Quick Chocolate Frosting (page 179) and a Dark Chocolate Cheesecake (page 180). These are recipes you can be proud to serve your guests at any dinner party.

Caramel Brownies

These are a bit thinner than the original, high-fat version, but they preserve the texture and full flavor. If you want a richer brownie, omit the low-fat sour cream and use 2 more tablespoons of butter; it will still have less than half the fat of the original recipe.

1 cup brown sugar, packed
2 tablespoons melted butter
2 tablespoons low-fat sour cream
½ cup Egg Beaters (or 2 eggs, beaten)
1 teaspoon vanilla

½ cup whole-wheat flour
½ teaspoon baking powder
⅛ teaspoon salt
¼ cup Grape-Nuts
¼ cup raisins

1. Put the brown sugar in a small mixing bowl and beat in the melted butter until smooth.
2. Add the sour cream and beat until well blended.
3. Add the Egg Beaters and vanilla and blend.
4. Sift the flour with the baking powder and salt.
5. Stir these ingredients into the egg mixture.
6. Add the Grape-Nuts and raisins and stir.
7. Pour into a lightly oiled 8×8×2-inch pan.
8. Bake at 350 degrees for about 25 minutes.
9. Cut when cool. ↦

16 brownies; serving size is 1 brownie.

Whole-Wheat Coffee Cake

BATTER

⅓ cup butter, softened

1 cup sugar

½ cup Egg Beaters (equivalent to 2 eggs)

1 teaspoon lemon juice

½ cup plain nonfat yogurt and ½ cup low-fat sour cream (try with 1 cup yogurt and no sour cream for a lower-fat version)

2 cups whole-wheat flour

1 teaspoon baking soda

½ teaspoon baking powder

1 teaspoon vanilla

TOPPING

½ cup brown sugar

2 teaspoons cinnamon

¼ cup each Grape-Nuts and raisins

1. Lightly oil a 9×13×2-inch baking pan.
2. Cream butter and sugar in a mixing bowl. Add the Egg Beaters and mix.
3. Stir the lemon juice into the yogurt/sour cream.
4. Combine the flour with the baking soda and baking powder.
5. Add the flour mixture to the butter/sugar mixture alternately with the yogurt/lemon juice mixture.
6. Stir in the vanilla and set aside.
7. Combine the topping ingredients and put a small amount in the bottom of the pan.
8. Layer in half the batter, top with half the remaining topping, add the remaining batter, and top with the remaining topping.
9. Bake at 300 degrees for about 45 minutes until cake tests done. ✤

24 servings.

Banana Muffins

1 cup oats

1 cup mashed ripe bananas (about 3 bananas)

⅔ cup plain fat-free yogurt

½ cup raisins

1 teaspoon vanilla

2 tablespoons corn oil

½ cup Egg Beaters

½ cup packed brown sugar

1½ cups whole-wheat flour

1 teaspoon baking powder

1 teaspoon baking soda

1 teaspoon cinnamon

¼ teaspoon salt

1. Preheat oven to 350 degrees.
2. Lightly oil a muffin tin or use paper muffin cups.
3. Mix the oats, mashed bananas, yogurt, raisins, and vanilla in a medium bowl.
4. Let stand 5 minutes.
5. In a small bowl, beat the oil and Egg Beaters with the brown sugar.
6. Beat the egg mix into the banana mixture.
7. Sift the flour with the baking powder, baking soda, cinnamon, and salt.
8. Add to the banana mixture and stir until just moistened.
9. Place in muffin cups and bake for 20–25 minutes.
10. Remove from oven and let cool.

12 muffins; serving size is 1 muffin.

Brownies

2 tablespoons butter, melted
1 cup sugar
3 tablespoons Neufchâtel cream cheese, softened
½ cup Egg Beaters (equivalent to 2 eggs)
1 teaspoon vanilla
½ cup whole-wheat flour
½ teaspoon baking powder
½ cup cocoa
½ cup Grape-Nuts

1. Preheat oven to 350 degrees.
2. In a small bowl, beat butter and sugar until blended.
3. Add the Neufchâtel and beat until smooth.
4. Add the Egg Beaters and vanilla and beat until well blended.
5. Sift the flour with the baking powder and add with the cocoa to the butter/sugar mixture. Mix just until all ingredients are blended.
6. Stir in the Grape-Nuts.
7. Oil an 8×8×2-inch baking pan and pour the brownie mixture into the pan, pushing to corners and sides.
8. Bake for 25 minutes and cut when cool.

16 brownies; serving size is 1 brownie.

Enid's Quick Fruit Pie

FILLING

2 cups any kind of fruit, cut into
   bite-size pieces
½ cup Egg Beaters
¼ cup sugar
2 tablespoons lemon juice

2 tablespoons plain nonfat
   yogurt
1 teaspoon vanilla
¼ teaspoon nutmeg (optional)

EASY CRUST (or you may use an already prepared crust)
1½ tablespoons melted butter
1 cup graham cracker crumbs

1. In a pie tin, combine butter with graham cracker crumbs and press onto
   the bottom and sides.
2. Bake in a 350-degree oven for 5–8 minutes until it just starts to brown.
3. Remove from oven and set aside.
4. When the crust has cooled slightly, place the fruit in it.
5. Combine all other ingredients except nutmeg and pour over the fruit.
6. Sprinkle with nutmeg if desired.
7. Bake at 350 degrees for 30 minutes.

8 servings.

Honey-Apricot Bread

1½ cups whole-wheat flour
⅔ cup firmly packed brown sugar
2½ teaspoons baking powder
½ teaspoon salt
1 teaspoon cinnamon
¼ teaspoon nutmeg
¼ cup Egg Beaters

1 cup skim or 1% milk
¼ cup honey
1 tablespoon butter, melted
1 cup bran flakes (your favorite
   brand)
1 cup dried apricots, finely
   chopped

1. Preheat oven to 350 degrees.
2. Mix the flour, sugar, baking powder, salt, and spices in a large bowl.
3. Beat the Egg Beaters in a small bowl and then stir in the milk, honey,
   and butter.
4. Add the wet ingredients to the dry and stir just until moistened (batter will be lumpy).

5. Stir in the cereal and apricots.
6. Pour into an 8×4×2½-inch loaf pan which has been sprayed with non-stick cooking spray.
7. Bake 55 to 60 minutes or until a toothpick inserted in the center comes out clean.
8. Cool 10 minutes and then remove from pan.
9. Cool completely on a wire rack.

Makes 16 (½-inch) slices; serving size is 1 slice.

Note: For easier slicing, wrap the bread in wax paper and store overnight at room temperature. ❧

Chewy Cocoa Cake
❧

1¾ cups sifted whole-wheat flour
1⅛ cups sugar
½ cup cocoa
1 teaspoon baking powder
1 teaspoon baking soda
¼ teaspoon salt
½ cup plain nonfat yogurt

4 tablespoons melted butter or margarine
¼ cup applesauce
1 teaspoon vanilla
¾ cup hot water
Quick Chocolate Frosting (below)

1. Preheat oven to 350 degrees.
2. Spray a 9×13×2-inch baking pan with non-stick cooking spray.
3. In a large bowl, stir together the first 6 ingredients.
4. Add the yogurt, butter, applesauce, vanilla, and water.
5. Beat on medium speed just until well blended.
6. Pour batter into the pan and bake for about 30 minutes or until a toothpick inserted in the center comes out dry.
7. Cool completely and then frost with Quick Chocolate Frosting. ❧

16 servings.

Quick Chocolate Frosting

1 teaspoon butter, softened
1½ cups powdered sugar
3 tablespoons cocoa

1 teaspoon vanilla
1½ to 2 tablespoons boiling water

1. Combine all ingredients except water.
2. Add water a little at a time, beating well, until desired consistency is achieved. ❧

Makes about ¾ cup.

Dark Chocolate Cheesecake

CRUST
1 cup zwieback crumbs
1 tablespoon brown sugar
1½ tablespoons melted butter or margarine

FILLING
1 pound firm tofu
16 ounces Neufchâtel cream
cheese
¾ cup Egg Beaters
⅔ cup cocoa
1 cup granulated white sugar
¾ cup firmly packed brown sugar

2 tablespoons cornstarch
1 cup low-fat sour cream
1 teaspoon vanilla
¼ cup Kahlua or other coffee
liqueur
Fresh strawberries (optional)

1. Preheat oven to 350 degrees. Combine the crumbs, brown sugar, and melted butter or margarine. Press firmly into the bottom of a 10-inch springform pan. Bake for 10 minutes, then set aside and let cool. Turn oven down to 300 degrees.
2. In a food processor or blender, beat the tofu until smooth and creamy. Mix with the Neufchâtel (8 ounces at a time) and beat until smooth.
3. In a separate bowl beat the eggs with the cocoa, sugars, and cornstarch.
4. Add the tofu/cheese mixture to the egg/cocoa mixture along with the sour cream, vanilla, and Kahlua. Beat until well blended.
5. Pour over the baked crust.

6. Bake for 1 hour to 1 hour and 15 minutes, or until the cake sets in the middle. Let the cake cool in the oven with the door slightly ajar for 2 hours.
7. Chill for at least 4 hours. Release sides of pan and garnish the cake with fresh sliced strawberries if desired.

24 servings.

Note: This cake can be sliced easily into 24 pieces by using a long strand of dental floss, of all things! ✏

Seasonings

Having a selection of your own favorite herbs and spices already mixed and ready to use is a great convenience. Think of the time you can save just reaching for a single jar and adding a single measure of a tried and tested blend, instead of having to select 4 to 6 different seasonings from your shelf each time you get ready to prepare dinner, and then having to carefully measure out the quantities. That extra bother alone can be enough to aggravate and discourage you when you're in a hurry.

Here are a few blends that I like. The garam masalas are better, I think, than any commercial curry I've ever tasted, and the Traditional Italian Herb Blend and Herb Salt are basic seasonings that you can use in Italian dishes and whenever a "generic" low-sodium herb mixture seems appropriate.

Garam Masala
✏

A "masala" is simply a mixture of spices. A "garam masala" is usually added to a dish late in the preparation or just before serving. However, I use one or another mix on poultry, rubbed into the skin or flesh before roasting after making a paste of my spices using a little oil and tamari (or soy sauce). I think you will find your mixtures more satisfying than any commercial curry ("curry" also just refers to a mixture of spices). Commonly used spices in garam masalas (or curries) are ginger, mustard seed, turmeric, cumin, black pepper, poppy seeds, fenugreek, fennel, mace, cloves, coriander, nutmeg, cardamom, cayenne pepper, cinnamon, and dried red chiles. Any 4 to 6 different ones will give your dishes a distinctive flavor. You will have noticed, perhaps, that we use a number of these spices in our recipes. Whenever possible, grind your own, but we have used powders (cinnamon) combined with seeds (cumin, coriander) ground with our mortar and pestle with excellent results. ∾

Simple Masalas
∾

In each of the following, just grind and combine spices (using seeds if available), or, if necessary, use pre-powdered versions. Depending upon how much you would like, consider a "part" to be either a tablespoon or a teaspoon. The mixtures will keep their flavor for several weeks in an airtight jar.

In the preparation of a given dish, you might like to try combining any one of these masalas with fresh garlic or ginger, minced or crushed, or garlic and onion powder. Add salt to taste.

  i. 2 parts cumin, 1 part cardamom, 1 part cloves

 ii. 3 parts cardamom, 3 parts cinnamon, 1 part cloves, 1 part cumin

iii. 4 parts black peppercorns, 4 parts coriander, 3 parts fennel, 1 part cloves, 1 part cardamom, 1 part cinnamon

 iv. 6 parts coriander, 6 parts dried red chiles, 1 part mustard, 1 part fenugreek, 1 part black peppercorns (this is a real hot one)

  v. 4 parts cumin, 2 parts powdered ginger, 2 parts turmeric, 1 part coriander, 1 part black peppercorns (try this on poultry; for a hot version, add 1 part cayenne pepper) ∾

Traditional Italian Herb Blend
∾

Basil is the perfect mate for tomatoes in Italian cooking. In fact, one of my favorite Italian chefs told me that he never adds any other herb to his tomato sauces. Of course, fresh basil lends food a wonderful flavor that cannot be reproduced from dried, just as the flavor of fresh garlic cannot be duplicated with the powder, but this blend will do nicely in a pinch. Try about a tablespoonful per quart of tomato sauce.

3 tablespoons dried basil leaves
1½ teaspoons garlic powder
1 teaspoon fresh-ground black pepper
½ teaspoon salt

Combine ingredients and store in an airtight container in a cool, dry place. ☙

Makes 4 tablespoons.

Herb Salt
☙

This is a general-purpose seasoning that can be used on vegetables (especially potatoes) and grains. If you haven't done much experimenting with herbs and spices in the past, you might find it fun to try mixing some formulas of your own. Store the mixture in a small herb jar just as you would any individual herb.

½ teaspoon dried basil
¼ teaspoon each thyme, dill weed, celery seed, dried parsley, and salt

Combine ingredients and grind together with mortar and pestle. ☙

Makes about 1¾ teaspoons.

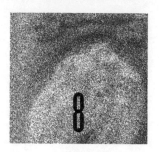

Pros and Cons of Nutrient and Herbal Supplementation

Should You Be Taking a Daily Multivitamin Pill?

Over 30 percent of the people in this country take some form of vitamin and mineral supplementation every day. At least another 10 percent do so on an occasional basis. In the absence of any clear health problems that would mandate taking some form of supplementation (for example, an iron deficiency in a premenopausal woman), most pill takers do it as a form of nutritional insurance. Some believe that it can make up for a lousy diet; others believe that our food supply is depleted of nutrients by modern agricultural methods; still others believe that dosing with antioxidant vitamins and minerals in pill form will prevent cancer and stop the aging process.

Probably nothing in the field of nutrition elicits more controversy among health professionals than the question of vitamin and mineral supplementation, or the value of herbal extracts and other dietary supplements, such as coenzyme Q10 and melatonin.

Looking first at the general question of vitamin and mineral supplementation, you can find, on the one hand, a health letter as prestigious as *Nutrition Action*, published by the Center for Science in the Public Interest, advising that everyone "take a multivitamin for insurance." The authors continue: "We can't prove that most people *need* to, but as long as you don't overdose or overpay or use it as an excuse to eat a lousy diet, you've got little to lose."[1] On the other hand, you can find the equally prestigious *Total Nutrition,* from the Mount Sinai School of Medicine, stating that supplements are "by definition unbalanced biochemistry" and "as likely to be harmful as to be helpful," followed by the opinion that they should be taken only on the advice of a responsible (and I hope knowledgeable[2]) health professional.[3]

The authors of these statements are respected and knowledgeable experts. They are all aware of the same research, yet feel compelled to issue completely different advice. Why such different decisions, and what exactly are the pros and cons?

ARGUMENTS FOR TAKING SUPPLEMENTS

There is a big difference in the arguments made for taking supplements between responsible health professionals, who have your welfare as their primary concern, and pseudo-experts, who have as their primary concern the marketing of certain products.

When responsible professionals believe that it's appropriate to recommend supplements as a form of nutritional insurance to the general public, they assume that the average person will not trouble to have a nutrition assessment and will not know whether they really have a need for supplementation. Therefore, they base their judgment and recommendation on certain facts:

1. While rare, instances of extreme deficiencies in certain nutrients are still seen in the United States. Since this is the case, then *marginal* deficiencies are certainly more widespread, and they may be making themselves seen in subtle ways. For example, fatigue, insomnia, headaches, irritability, lethargy, loss of appetite, or general malaise, while usually from other causes, may, in fact, be early behavioral or psychological signs of a developing or ongoing marginal deficiency in one or another of a number of different nutrients.

2. While almost all healthy people can meet their needs from a varied, nu-

[1]"Vitamin Smarts," cover story by Bonnie Liebman, M.S., and David Schardt, *Nutrition Action,* Vol. 22, No. 5, November 1995.

[2]On a day when I was working on this chapter I received a critical call from a person who had read in one of my articles that prolonged use of aspirin might impair folate status. Her doctor had told her that he was not aware of any such interaction.

[3]"What Is a Healthy Food Plan?," Chapter 1 by Victor Herbert, M.D., and Tracy Stopler Kasdan, M.S., R.D., in *Total Nutrition: The Only Guide You'll Ever Need,* edited by Victor Herbert, M.D., F.A.C.P., and Genell J. Subak-Sharpe, M.S. (New York: St. Martin's Press, 1995).

tritious diet, *many* people, out of distaste or disinclination, are eating unbalanced diets and may be omitting entire food groups. As I mentioned earlier, almost half the people in the United States eat no fruit on a given day and 1 out of 4 people skip vegetables. Only 9 percent of the population consumes the minimal amount of fruits and vegetables recommended by the USDA in the Food Pyramid guide to sound nutrition. In one of the nutrition research projects with students at Vanderbilt that I conducted before my retirement from the university I found students who ate only one piece of fruit a week.

3. Some people, in special circumstances, may find it hard to obtain the nutrition they need from food alone. These include women who bleed excessively during menstruation, women who are pregnant or breast feeding, people with low calorie intakes (some of whom, for one reason or another, including illness, simply can't eat enough to obtain adequate nourishment), and certain vegetarians (called vegans) who exclude all animal products from their diets, including milk, cheese, and eggs.[4]

4. Because of the above considerations, some experts feel that it is reasonable to make a general recommendation to take a supplement, *as long as the supplement does not exceed the amounts of the various nutrients that a person might consume by eating a nutritious diet.* Thus, they will recommend that you find a "balanced" supplement that approximates the Recommended Daily Allowances (RDAs, sometimes called Daily Values, or DVs).[5]

5. Finally, some experts have felt that the evidence, while inconsistent, is strong enough to merit a recommendation to take supplements of certain antioxidants, such as vitamins C and E and beta-carotene, in quantities that exceed the amounts that a person might consume from food on a daily basis, in the hope that they might help protect against heart disease and cancer. The more cautious recommendations have been to take amounts such as 250–500 milligrams of vitamin C, 200–400 international units (IU) of vitamin E, and 15,000–25,000 IU of beta-carotene. While some experts were suggesting two or three times these amounts, the more cautious recommendations were thought to be harmless and at levels that just might do some good. However, a re-

[4]The issue with vegans is the likelihood of a vitamin B_{12} deficiency. Vegans need to make sure they find a source of active B_{12} either through fortification of certain foods, such as soy milk and meat replacements, or through supplements.

[5]The article from *Nutrition Action* that I referred to in Footnote 1 points out that it is quite difficult to find a supplement that meets this requirement. The authors make some useful suggestions for persons who try to follow their advice.

cent study showed that as little as 50 IU of vitamin E may increase the risk of hemorrhagic stroke, and another study showed an increase in the risk of lung cancer among smokers who took beta-carotene.[6]

The pseudo-experts who have a marketing interest make far different claims to entice the public to buy vitamin and mineral supplements. They will go to the limits of the law, and frequently beyond until stopped, in trying to frighten you into buying their products or in making extravagant, unproven claims about their miraculous powers.

Pseudo-experts often start by making claims that a person needs to obtain some optimum amount of certain vitamins and minerals every single day. They also may claim that our plant foods are lacking vitamins and minerals because modern agricultural practices have depleted the soil in which they are grown of essential nutrients. They may claim you need supplementation because, if you buy your vegetables and fruits at the supermarket and they have been grown with the use of commercial fertilizers, they will be lacking in the nutrients that are supplied by 100 percent organic methods. None of these things is true, as I will explain more fully in the next section of this chapter. Perhaps most insidious is the claim that nutrients in food are no longer adequate to protect us against the dangers of an increasingly polluted environment. While pollution is a real danger, I know of no proof that vitamin and mineral supplementation can help protect us from it, in either the presence or absence of a nutritious diet.

Those who have an interest in selling you something may base their claims on anything from a single study that managed to find its way into the research literature, though no one else has ever been able to replicate this finding, to a single customer's enthusiastic report, calling this the result of a "clinical study." Sometimes, as in the first example I'm about to give, the product they are pushing actually does contain substances found in foods that protect against cancer and heart disease, and which have shown disease-preventing or disease-limiting activity when extracted from these foods and used in laboratory studies with animals. *But there is no evidence that the pills they are selling contain the substances in the amounts, relationships, or chemical forms that would be helpful to any particular individual or to entire unselected groups of people in fighting disease.*

[6]Many health professionals have been encouraging smokers to supplement with at least 100 milligrams of vitamin C daily because smoking depletes the body's supply of this important antioxidant. My recommendation is to consume extra citrus fruit, rather than a supplement, since the citrus fruit will contain at least another hundred different phytochemicals that may have protective functions equally as important as the vitamin C.

Here, from my files, is a short list of some claims used in merchandising materials to encourage you to purchase supplements, for which I can find no proof:

1. A "super antioxidant" capsule containing "a wholly balanced formula" of vitamins A (from beta-carotene), C, E, calcium, zinc, selenium, N-acetyl-cysteine, L-glutathione, alfalfa juice and wheat sprout concentrates in a base of rosemary, citrus bioflavonoids, and green tea will help "[d]estroy the free radicals that damage cells; provide excellent support for the body's immune system, making it an effective disease preventative; protect cells against premature, abnormal aging; promote the growth of healthy cells."
2. "Lysine and vitamin C can 'scour' arteries clean and eliminate angina pain." (Lysine is an essential amino acid once touted as a cure for both oral and genital herpes, which it isn't.)
3. Vitamin C in a special blend of vitamins and minerals can "reverse 'irreversible' cataracts."
4. "Magnesium can help prevent—and even REVERSE—serious asthma attacks where drugs often fail."
5. Glucosamine sulfate is "a natural remedy that's 30 times more effective than any drug on the market" in treating arthritis.
6. Chromium picolinate turns "wobbly, unattractive fat into lean, new muscle—with no exercise required."
7. Magnesium and vitamin B_6 can "stop kidney stones forever."
8. "You can grow smarter, sharper, and even boost your IQ as you grow older," with a special combination of vitamins and minerals (vitamins C, A, B complex, and trace minerals) whose formula you can only get by purchasing certain materials from the merchandiser.

Finally, I think it's important to point out that while vitamins and minerals, when found in foods at or around the RDA levels, can promote health and well-being, when taken in pills at higher, megadose levels, they can be toxic and even deadly. For example, cases of liver damage have now been reported at what experts previously thought was a safe level of 25,000 IU daily of vitamin A. And while all the antioxidant vitamins, minerals, and phytochemicals that I've been talking about may protect against cancer and heart disease when consumed in real food, *at higher levels their biochemical activity changes and they may actually promote cancer and other illnesses.* That is, antioxidants can become oxidants when you take too much of them. Which brings me to the arguments against supplementation.

ARGUMENTS AGAINST TAKING SUPPLEMENTS

First, the general argument. Those who argue in general against taking supplements without professional advice based on a nutritional assessment that has shown a specific need point out that real food contains a *balanced* biochemistry of nutrients and phytochemicals. There are hundreds of them in any given food. The nutrients and phytochemicals come in different chemical forms (that is, any individual vitamin or phytochemical can have more than one chemical form, each slightly different and each active in a different way). Supplements contain only a fraction of these nutrients and phytochemicals, and they do not contain the different chemical variations—they are *unbalanced* biochemistry. For this reason, experts who argue against them believe that supplements are as likely to harm some people as they are to help others.

They also point out that people do not have to eat a perfect diet every day because the body stores enough of all vitamins and minerals to last several weeks, if not months, without the appearance of any physical deficiency. This holds true even for the water-soluble vitamins such as C and the B complex, which those who want to sell supplements would have you believe must be eaten (or supplemented) at least at RDA levels on a daily basis. Of course, this does not mean that you can stay in the best of health by omitting an essential nutrient for extended periods of time, but that your diet must be varied enough over a period of days to provide the essentials, for example, a week at a time.

One of the most telling arguments against the value of supplementation is that it has no effect on overall mortality among Americans: a recent study conducted by researchers at the U.S. Centers for Disease Control and published in the *American Journal of Public Health* (April 1993) found that those who do not take supplements live just as long as those who do. This is what you might expect if some supplement takers were helped, others harmed, and a majority not affected at all.

Another argument against supplementation is that there are a whole host of nutrient interactions, some facilitating, some interfering. One well-known example of both facilitation and interference with respect to a single important target nutrient is the facilitation of iron absorption by vitamin C, but the reduction in iron absorption by calcium and phosphorus. The facilitation of iron absorption by vitamin C is in itself double-edged because, while it can be helpful to some, too much vitamin C (for example, even 1 gram) can mobilize so much iron as to cause serious harm in others.

Lesser-known examples of interference, possibly important in the prevention of cancer and heart disease, are the reduction in absorption of other carotenoids when large quantities of beta-carotene are present, and a depression in the absorption of copper when large quantities of vitamin C are present. This is of special interest because copper is an essential constituent of a very important antioxidant enzyme called superoxide dismutase, which protects cell membranes from free-radical damage. Thus, with either beta-carotene or vitamin C, if you take supplements, you can be taking in so much that you turn a good thing into a bad one. You may be interfering with the activity of other equally essential good things, such as other carotenoids and the body's production of its own army of antioxidants.

The examples of important interactions that I have just given are but a few among the scores that are already well known to nutritional biochemists, and which form the basis for one of the arguments against supplementation. Researchers feel that known interactions may represent only the tip of the iceberg—there may be scores of others equally as important as, or even more important than, those already recognized.

Finally, I know of no objective evidence that foods are becoming less nutritious as a result of modern agricultural methods. If plants don't get the nutrients they need from the soil, or can't convert the substances they do take in from the soil into the chemical forms they can use, they don't grow. Plants manufacture the same substances when encouraged by either organic or commercial fertilizers. And while it is true that the mineral content of the soil will affect the mineral content of a plant and certain soils may be low in essential minerals (for example, selenium and iodine in certain regions), we are highly unlikely to suffer any deficiencies as a result because the fruits, vegetables, and grain foods we find in our supermarkets are grown in many different soils in different sections of the United States and other parts of the world.

Herbal Mania: Facts and Fantasies

The controversy over the risks and benefits of using herbal supplements exceeds even that surrounding the value of vitamin and mineral supplementation. Part of the reason for this is that very little research on the subject has been done in the tradition of Western medicine, with appropriate control over dosages and with experimental designs that allow elimination of competing explanations for positive findings. The evidence in favor is almost entirely anecdotal, and even though it may be the accumulation of hundreds of years of testimony, since most illnesses are self-limiting any positive results cannot be attributed to an herbal remedy with any certainty. In addition, persons with a vested interest in promoting herbal remedies rarely point to any negative findings, including possible toxic reactions. Perhaps even more telling is that much of the evidence one way or the other may be based on misidentification of the actual herbs used in the first place.

If you have a serious interest in the use of herbs and herbal extracts as preventives or remedies, I think you need to be aware of several circumstances that make it very difficult to make informed decisions and dependable choices among the many herbal products being touted in today's burgeoning market. At the very top of the list is that, thanks to the Dietary Supplement and Health Education Act passed by Congress in 1994, virtually all regulations that might ensure efficacy, the truth of any claims regarding that efficacy, and the safety and quality of herbal products have been wiped out.

What this really means is that you have no assurance that two bottles of the same herbal preparation from the same manufacturer are actually the same in content or potency, or that a preparation from a different source, claiming to have the same potency on the packaging, really does have the same potency. While the 1994 act calls for some standards to be set in the future, such standards have not been clearly defined, and whatever they end up being they are at least two years away. The truth of the matter is, as much as we might dislike government red tape and interference, Congress has made the FDA virtually powerless when it comes to protecting the public from both fraud and danger with respect to herbal products and other kinds of supplements. Because of this situation, it's truly a "buyer beware" market out there.

Let me give just a few examples.

In order to keep abreast of developments in alternative medicine I subscribed last year to a newsletter on that subject. As a result of this subscription my name found its way onto a mailing list distributed to other writers and publishers of materials having to do with nontraditional remedies and to manufacturers of such remedies. Here are just three samples of what I found in a recently arrived full-color, 26-page advertisement for one of these other newsletters which carried the blazing headline "Medically-Proven MIRACLES OF HEALING CENSORED By The Medical Establishment" (the word "censored" in bright red) and which promised, immediately beneath, to tell me about "the stunning, no-side-effects cures that greedy drug companies and FDA bureaucrats don't want you to have":

1. Coenzyme Q10 "has such miraculous, heart-healing properties it could someday make heart disease extinct."

    While this substance has antioxidant properties and is involved in energy metabolism, it is produced by the body itself in every cell, and, since enzymes and other substances taken by mouth are digested and chemically transformed into other substances, researchers really don't know if Q10 works the same when swallowed as when produced in your body cells.[7]

2. Gugulipid (an herbal extract) "can lower cholesterol counts up to 27% in just four weeks."

    This claim is based on the results of a study done in India and published in 1989 in the *Journal of the Association of Physicians of India*. While the extract may have a modest impact on cholesterol, the average reduction in the controlled phase of the study was not 27 percent, but 11 percent, and a number of participants did not respond to gugulipid therapy.

3. The healing properties of ginseng are being ignored "despite the fact that over 1,000 clinical studies have confirmed its undeniable power to increase your stamina, boost your energy levels and supercharge your resistance."

    There's been more hype and hoax over the powers of ginseng during the past several years than with any other herbal product. *Results in human studies are completely equivocal.* When you buy ginseng you should be aware that (a) there are a number of different species, (b) other plants are similar and often confused with ginseng, (c) many preparations labeled as ginseng may contain no ginseng at all, (d) when they do contain ginseng, the presence of the supposedly active ingredients (ginsenosides) in capsules may vary up to 20-fold from capsule to capsule, and (e) the preparations may contain other ingredients, including stimulants, such as caffeine. Of course, as I have pointed out, many of these problems are due to the almost complete lack of regulations governing the production of herbal products.

The advertisement goes on to tout, in greatly exaggerated terms, the value of other herbal preparations, some of which may prove to be useful, including saw palmetto, feverfew, and milk thistle. While my focus in this book is on the prevention of cancer and heart disease, because of the rapidly growing interest in herbal preventives and remedies I have in-

---

[7]Another marketer of this product claims that "most of us, due to bad diet, lack of exercise and the stress of everyday life have severe deficiencies of this essential coenzyme."

cluded a summary of the potential uses and dangers for some of the most important herbs and other supplements, including recent fads such as melatonin (see Table 8.1, pages 197–99).

HERBS AS PREVENTIVES OF CARDIOVASCULAR DISEASE AND CANCER

Since about 25 percent of all drugs prescribed in this country derive their active ingredient from plants, since several are being used in the treatment of heart disease and cancer (for example, digitalis for congestive heart failure, vinblastine and vincristine for many different cancers), and since so many different plant foods contain phytochemicals that may protect against heart disease and cancer, it certainly seems reasonable to expect that herbs and spices would contain similar beneficial substances. And there are some that do, but there is the frequent problem of separating the hype from reality.[8]

Cardiovascular Disease. At the top of the list in the prevention of atherosclerotic heart disease is GARLIC! And, of course, you have heard this before. It's been used as a food and medicine for thousands of years. A great many well-done studies have affirmed its usefulness, together with that of other members of the genus *Allium,* including onions, leeks, chives, and shallots (although to a lesser degree).

The active ingredient in garlic that protects against cardiovascular disease is allicin, which is formed when a garlic clove is crushed. Allicin appears to perform a number of useful functions in the circulatory system that can protect against heart disease: it helps lower cholesterol, inhibits platelet aggregation, and increases fibrinolytic activity. These last two activities keep the blood from getting too sticky and clotting.

While there is some disagreement on the exact amount of garlic a person needs to obtain a beneficial effect, most authorities suggest eating at least one fresh clove (weight about 4 grams) a day. The active ingredient is formed during chewing. Unfortunately, garlic powder is not as effective as the fresh clove since the formation of the active ingredient, allicin,

---

[8]In the discussion that follows I have checked my own search of the medical literature with the information provided in two excellent books written for the lay person by Varro E. Tyler, Ph.D., Sc.D., Distinguished Professor of Pharmacognosy at Purdue University and one of America's leading authorities on plants and their medicinal uses. They are *The Honest Herbal: A Sensible Guide to the Use of Herbs and Related Remedies* and *Herbs of Choice: The Therapeutic Use of Phytomedicinals,* both published by Pharmaceutical Products Press (1993 and 1994, respectively). I highly recommend these two books to anyone interested in the use of herbs as preventives, remedies, or adjuncts to the medical treatment of any illness.

is prevented by the acids in the stomach. So, if you want to avoid eating garlic cloves, crushed or otherwise, you must take a commercial product. Tablets or capsules made from a powder require a special low temperature in drying to preserve the active ingredient. In addition, they must have an enteric coating that will allow them to pass through the stomach without dissolving and reach the small intestine intact, where the alkaline environment will allow the formation of the active ingredient. The potency of any commercial garlic product (other than raw garlic) is really uncertain since the activity of allicin may be lost when alcohol or water is used in preparation or the garlic is in an oil base. In fact, the Center for Science in the Public Interest has tested a number of different brands of garlic pills and found a 40-fold variation in the active ingredient.

With all of the complications I've just enumerated, it's obvious that "fresh is best." Indeed, fresh garlic appears to be one of nature's most valuable foods: other research has found it to be of benefit in the treatment of digestive disorders, bacterial and fungal infections, and hypertension, as well as cancer (which I'll discuss in a moment).

Among other herbs that appear to be useful in the prevention and treatment of cardiovascular diseases are hawthorn and *Ginkgo biloba*. Standardized extracts of hawthorn, not available in the United States, are widely used in Europe for mild conditions of angina.[9] Similarly, a standardized extract of *Ginkgo biloba* is widely used for a variety of peripheral vascular disorders, including cerebral circulatory disturbances (for example, reduced functional capacity that manifests itself in symptoms such as vertigo, tinnitus, and memory problems) and intermittent claudication (cramping pain in the calves brought on by walking short distances). In Europe the extract (GBE) is an approved drug and the contents of the different forms (tablets and liquids, including intravenous forms) are stan-

---

[9]The German government has set up a commission (Commission E) to evaluate the safety and efficacy of herbal products. Absolute certainty of safety and reasonable certainty of efficacy are requirements before any product can be marketed. Commission E relies on a large body of data gathered from all available sources for its information. Whereas the FDA requires extensive and expensive clinical trials, Commission E accepts case studies and documented medical experience as well, when the results of extensive clinical trials are not available. Using its approach, Commission E has compiled the most complete and reliable information about herbal medicinals that exists in the world today. The U.S. government, by requiring extensive clinical trials, has made the approval of phytomedicinals much more costly and has prevented their standardization and availability in this country to the same extent as in Europe. Since herbs grow freely and are not patentable, no drug company can make a profitable investment doing the kind of research it would take to prove their safety and efficacy as drugs by present FDA standards (it can cost a couple of hundred million dollars). Many authorities in the United States are recommending that we adopt the approach being used in Germany.

dardized, whereas in the United States GBE is sold as a food supplement, without the same standards of quality control.

While on the subject of circulatory diseases, it's worth noting that also available and approved in Europe, but not in the United States, are preparations made from horse-chestnut seeds that are used with some apparent success to treat venous insufficiency and varicosities. These include forms that can be taken orally, as well as ointments and liniments.

While all of the above herbal preparations contain representatives from the same classes of phytochemicals that occur in fruits and vegetables, some of them are in forms that appear to be unique to a particular species. It is unfortunate that research is not available to determine what, if anything, their consumption can add to the health benefits of a nutritious diet.

Cancer. A number of plants have supplied us with potent drugs for fighting established cancers (for example, catharanthus for vinblastine and vincristine, podophyllum for etoposide, and the Pacific yew for taxol), and in Table 3.1 (pages 27–29) I listed a number of herbs that have shown protective effects either in epidemiological studies or in laboratory research, including garlic, basil, parsley, and rosemary. However, I know of no objective research that convincingly demonstrates that commercial supplements of these or other herbs, in amounts over and above what you might use in normal food preparation, can contribute to the prevention of cancer. Nevertheless, many claims are made for herbs that might increase resistance to stress (which can lower resistance and may play a role in the development of infections as well as cancer and cardiovascular disease) and for herbs that may stimulate and support the body's own immune system in resisting disease.

Both the true ginsengs of the genus *Panax* and eleuthero (known as "Siberian ginseng" but not a ginseng at all) have gotten reputations as tonics or "adaptogens," meaning that they can help build resistance to stress of all origins and contribute to a feeling of physical and mental well-being and vitality. I have already mentioned some considerable problems involved with the use of these herbs. While there is a good deal of research with animals that supports their reputation as adaptogens, there is little with humans, and there is no evidence that they might have any preventive powers with respect to cancer.

Echinacea, on the other hand, does appear to act as an immunostimulant, increasing the release of interferon and tumor necrosis factor, both of which, theoretically, might interfere with the development of cancer. However, there is no direct evidence that extracts of echinacea actually do interfere with the development of cancer in the human body. Nevertheless, there are confirmed uses for echinacea, and in Europe it is employed as a supportive measure (that is, in combination with other drugs) in the treatment of respiratory and urinary tract infections and hard-to-heal wounds. There is also some evidence that echinacea might be effective in preventing or treating the common cold. Experts in the field agree that this herb deserves further study.

Recently, certain ingredients in Indian spice blends (garam masalas), such as turmeric, have been found to have anti-tumor potency in test tube and animal studies, as has a Chinese and Japanese herbal concoction known as Xiao Chaihu Tang in China and Sho-saiko-to in Japan. This latter concoction, made from bupleurum (hare's ear root), scutellaria (skullcap), ginseng, pinellia tuber (half summer), licorice, ginger, and jujube (red date), has a long reputation as a folk remedy for liver cancer. However, as you will note in my recipes for garam masalas, there is no such thing as a standard formula, and when I compared formulas for the Chinese/Japanese herbal concoction in different sources, I discovered a similar situation. Based on other research reports, licorice may prove to be the most active beneficial ingredient in the mixture, but there is also evidence that scutellaria (skullcap), as well as licorice, may be toxic and actually *cause* liver damage or become carcinogenic. It's a question of dosage, and at this point information about beneficial versus harmful dosages is not available.

With this bit of information I return to emphasize the warnings I gave earlier in this chapter about the use of herbal supplements: There is no guarantee of safety and no reasonable assurance of efficacy when you purchase commercial herbal preparations in this country. That's not to say that there are no safe and effective herbs. But because there is no pressure on producers to conform to certain quality, effectiveness, and safety standards, the field is overflowing with hype and fraud. While certain herbal preparations may, in the future, be found capable of making unique contributions to the prevention of heart disease and cancer, and regulations may be passed that would help assure that you're getting what you expect to get and pay for in a supplement, right now your best assurance is to eat the kind of plant-rich diet I have been encouraging you to consume and to include liberal amounts of garlic and the other herbs I've listed in Table 3.1 *in exactly the form in which you can buy them in your supermarket.*

For your general information, I have listed the possible (but often not proven) benefits and risks (when known) of a number of popular herbs and supplements in Table 8.1. All of those with potential benefits deserve further study, but at the present time I would not recommend that you "self-medicate" with any of them. However, if your personal health situ-

Table 8.1 POTENTIAL VALUE AND DANGERS OF VARIOUS HERBAL AND OTHER DIETARY SUPPLEMENTS

Supplement	Potential Value	Dangers
Chamomile	Combats indigestion; anti-inflammatory (internally as tea, externally as oil or ointment); antispasmotic (suppression of muscle spasms and menstrual cramps).	People with allergies to ragweed, asters, chrysanthemums, and others in the daisy family should use caution.
Chaparral	Conflicting evidence that one of its ingredients, nordihydroguaiaretic acid, may inhibit progression of cancer.	**DANGER:** Cases of acute liver disease have been reported. The FDA does not consider it safe for human consumption; watch out for it as an ingredient in other herbal preparations.
Comfrey	May aid in treatment of ulcers and healing of wounds.	**DANGER:** Serious liver damage and danger to kidneys, lungs, and gastrointestinal tract.
Chromium picolinate	Promoted for weight loss.	**DANGER:** heart arrhythmias, possible chromosome damage, and cancer risk.
Coenzyme Q10	May strengthen the heart and increase longevity; antioxidant properties.	Uncertain effectiveness when swallowed, but apparently no reported side effects.
Echinacea	May increase resistance to and lessen severity of colds and stimulate immune system.	As with chamomile, persons allergic to flowers in the daisy family should use caution.
Ephedra (ma huang)	Contains ephedrine and promoted for weight loss and as an energy booster; useful in treatment of nasal congestion and asthma; may be combined with caffeine in supplements.	**DANGER:** Elevates blood pressure; may cause heart palpitations, nerve injury, and stroke.
Feverfew	May be useful in prevention and treatment of migraine headaches.	Labeled potency of commercial tablets may be unreliable; chewing leaves may cause mouth sores.
Garlic	Helps lower cholesterol and blood pressure; may protect against cancer; antibacterial; best source is raw.	Commercial preparations are of unreliable potency. Persons on anticoagulants should check with their doctors since the dosage may need reducing.

Table 8.1 POTENTIAL VALUE AND DANGERS OF VARIOUS HERBAL AND OTHER DIETARY SUPPLEMENTS (*continued*)

Supplement	Potential Value	Dangers
Ginger	May help prevent motion sickness and nausea from other causes.	No reported toxic effects but very large overdoses may inhibit blood clotting and cause cardiac arrhythmias.
Gingko biloba	Circulatory aid that increases blood flow to the brain and may improve concentration and memory; may alleviate headaches and tinnitus. May help relieve leg cramps.	Overdoses can cause diarrhea, nausea, and vomiting. May interfere with action of anticoagulants.
Ginseng	May increase resistance to stress, increase stamina, boost the immune system.	Equivocal results in human studies. Uncertain potency and quality of herbal preparations, but apparently little or no toxicity.
Hawthorn	Dilates blood vessels, lowers blood pressure, reduces tendency to angina by relaxing the heart muscle.	While toxicity is low, this herb should be used in consultation with a physician since self-treatment for something as deadly as heart disease can be dangerous.
Lobelia (Indian tobacco)	Like nicotine, can both stimulate and then depress the central nervous system. It was once used in the treatment of asthma and chronic bronchitis.	**DANGER:** Can interfere with breathing, reduce blood pressure, and induce rapid heart rate; may lead to convulsions; can be lethal in large doses.
Melatonin	May be effective in relief of insomnia and treatment of jet lag. Claims for cancer and longevity unproven.	Occasional side effects include grogginess, mild depression, and low sex drive. Long-term effects unknown.
Milk thistle	May protect liver against various toxins that help prevent and treat cirrhosis and hepatitis.	No toxic effects have so far been reported. Self-treatment for liver ailments is not advised and use should be under the supervision of a physician.
Saw palmetto	Used in benign prostate hypertrophy (BPH) to improve urinary flow.	May have a sedative effect. (The effective ingredient in saw palmetto requires extraction by hexane or alcohol; preparations

Supplement	Potential Value	Dangers
		with the intended use for BPH are illegal in this country.)
Shark cartilage	Cancer preventive.	No proof of efficacy, but apparently no reported side effects.
Valerian	Mild sedative and tranquilizer.	No significant side effects have been noted.

ation might benefit from their use—that is, if you are at high risk for or are actually suffering from some degenerative disease—I suggest you seek out a physician or other knowledgeable health professional who will search for the best combination of traditional medications as well as phytomedicinals to meet your individual needs. In certain circumstances there may, in fact, be one pill worth considering by many people, on the advice of their physician, and that is aspirin.

Aspirin contains a member of a class of compounds called salicylates found in many plants, for example, willow and birch bark, and wintergreen. Some of these compounds are naturally anti-inflammatory, thin the blood slightly, and help prevent blood clots. The form that is synthesized as aspirin, that is, acetylsalicylic acid, is particularly effective in these actions and several studies show that it may help prevent heart attacks in susceptible persons. Recent research has shown that it may help prevent colon cancer, as well. The dosage recommended in most cases is either half an aspirin a day or one every other day. (Gastrointestinal irritation is rare, but may occur even at this low concentration of the drug, and some people can react with hives and asthma.)

Recommendations

I have just made a recommendation with regard to herbal supplements and aspirin, but the question remains what is the best course of action with respect to vitamins and minerals.

When you follow the Cancer Prevention Good Health Diet there is very little likelihood that vitamin and mineral supplementation can contribute anything more to your health or add to your longevity. If anything, socking yourself everyday with an unvarying dose of a certain limited number of nutrients may lead to imbalances. For example, I mentioned earlier the facilitation of iron absorption by vitamin C and the blocking action on iron by calcium and phosphorus. There are scores of such interactions. In a varied, nutritious diet, from day to day, the amount of facilitation and blocking action will vary and balance out over time. With a constant, continual hit at the same daily level of one or more nutrients via a supplement, the balancing may be less likely. Similarly, a high intake of one compound in a certain class may depress absorption or activity of other similar compounds, as in the case of beta-carotene versus the other carotenoids. This presents an unknown but possibly important danger.

But suppose you don't eat a balanced diet—for example, you are one of those Americans who has no fruit and skips vegetables on a number of days during a given week. Will a so-called balanced vitamin and mineral supplement at or near the RDAs (which are close to what you might consume in a healthful diet of those particular nutrients) give you any kind of insurance? The most "balanced" supplement that I have examined contained 31 of the 50-plus essential nutrients, and none of the hundreds of other phytochemicals that may also prove to be essential in the prevention of degenerative diseases. What some experts refer to as "balanced supplements" remain *biochemically unbalanced nutrition.*

While most responsible health professionals oppose the use of megadoses of any vitamin or mineral by normal, healthy people (they may have a place after surgery or as adjunctive therapy in certain illnesses), many support the general use of supplements at the RDAs because they feel they can do no harm and may offer some insurance. However, that insurance is not needed by people who consume a nutritious diet. Obviously, for people whose diets are so lacking and unbalanced that they are in danger of a deficiency disease such as scurvy, pellagra, or beriberi, supplementation is called for. But for the average American who is eating the typical, unbalanced American diet, supplementation is still chemically unbalanced and does not substitute for eating a nutritious diet. It may do as much harm to some individuals as it does good for others.

So let me encourage you once again to take stock of your current situation because there is no substitute for a balanced, nutritious diet based primarily on plant foods, such as I have outlined for you here. It's your best shot at reducing your odds of developing cancer and heart disease.

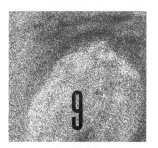

Beyond Diet

PHYSICAL ACTIVITY, MANAGING STRESS, AND REDUCING THE HEALTH DANGERS IN YOUR ENVIRONMENT

The Cancer Prevention Good Health Diet lays the cornerstone on which you can complete the building of a healthful lifestyle. The other building blocks include physical activity, managing stress, and reducing the dangers to your health in your home and work environments.

Physical Activity

Do you perform most of your work in a sitting position? If so, and if you haven't found a way to include some recreational physical activity in your daily life, you qualify as a "sedentary person."

Most health-conscious people are aware that lack of physical activity is an important risk factor for heart disease and hypertension as well as for obesity. Experts estimate that lack of activity contributes to the premature deaths of about 250,000 Americans a year! Adding 40 to 60 minutes of whole-body movement each day, *of almost any kind,* can reduce the risk of cardiovascular disease and usually results in weight loss in overweight people. What is not as well known is that daily physical activity may also play a significant role in cancer prevention.

HOW PHYSICAL ACTIVITY MAY HELP PROTECT
AGAINST CANCER

Moderate physical activity helps protect against cancer in several ways. It enhances the strength and activity of various components of the immune system and, as numerous studies have shown, may help reduce the risk of many cancers, including colon cancer (by stimulating bowel movement), prostate cancer in men (by possibly lowering levels of testosterone), and breast, uterine, and ovarian cancer in women (by helping to regulate estrogen production, body weight, and body-fat distribution).

What I'm talking about is *moderate activity*. All physical activity promotes the formation of free radicals, but *intense* physical activity, such as marathon running and training, may produce more than the body can deal with effectively. Research shows that after a marathon race, runners' immune systems are weakened and they may become more susceptible to infection. *Moderate activity*, however, builds the immune system and increases resistance to disease. As usual, with physical activity as in so many aspects of our lives, more is not always better—moderation is the key.

So the questions are: What is a healthful level of physical activity, and how can you fit it into what may already be an overly busy schedule?

THE PHYSICAL-ACTIVITY GOAL

If you sit for a living, you probably are on your feet, moving about, for less than an hour a day. When people in sedentary jobs wear pedometers, they find that they walk only about 2 miles during their entire waking hours. That's about 4 or 5 miles less than humans moved about each day, for thousands of years, before the advent of electricity in our homes, refrigeration, automobiles, elevators, and so on. If you are a sedentary person, keep track. You, too, may be amazed to find that you are spending 23 hours a day either sitting or lying down. And if you feel lethargic, perhaps even moderately depressed without an apparent cause, lack of physical activity may be the reason.

Your body was made for moving. Before the technological advances that have occurred during the last 100 years, which have turned us into couch potatoes, humans had to perform many hours of manual labor each day just to get the job of living done. As a result of thousands of years of evolution our bodies adapted well to these demands, and we suffer when we don't exercise our capacities. To be in the best physical and mental condition, you must find a way to restore the level of activity that your body was designed for. And as I said, just about any kind of movement will do, as long as you move your entire body (as in walking or swimming or other active sports) or the major muscles (as in bicycling). House cleaning and outdoor work, such as gardening, also qualify if done in an energetic fashion!

How can you find a way to get active?

Basically, there are two approaches:

1: If the idea of building a 40- to 60-minute period of physical activity into your day is either unappealing or impossible, find a way to get up and walk about for 5 minutes on the hour. Walk corridors, climb steps, do deep knee bends, stretch, rotate your arms. Not only will this add up to the equivalent of between 2 and 3 miles of walking, but it will relax and refresh you. You are likely to find that break periods of this kind contribute to productivity and creativity in your work, whatever you do.

There may be certain benefits to this periodic approach if you are concerned with weight management. A recent study found that people who scheduled their exercise in several 10-minute periods each day rather than in one long session were more likely to meet their goal, exercise more, and lose more weight.

Whether you aim for 5 or 10 minutes, getting up and moving about on the hour is an especially important relaxation strategy if you work at a computer or in any other job that requires repetitive movements of your arms, hands, and fingers in a sitting position. In addition, pressure of the upper body on the lower back while sitting for a long stretch of time can lead to the development of back problems, and it is certainly not good for the circulation in your legs. So stretch and stand tall to relieve the back pressure when you get up to walk around. To increase circulation, go as briskly as you can, without hurting yourself, and, if it's convenient, climb one or two flights of stairs.

2: I must admit that my own personal preference for activity is for the longer periods. If you can find a way to build up to 40 to 60 minutes of some kind of brisk activity each day, from walking to an active sport, or some mixture, I think you will experience some special psychological as well as physical benefits. It's something very hard to describe in words—but once you do experience it, you will know what I mean. If you have been a sedentary person, you will begin to think of yourself as an active person. Besides all the long-term health benefits that may lie in store for you 20, 30, 40, or more years in the future, you will immediately feel stronger and more vigorous, physically and mentally. These changes will have an impact on your self-concept—you will like yourself better!

Many people find that companionship is important if they consider starting a walking program, and of course it's essential to find congenial opponents or teammates when you embark on an active sport.

Sometimes making an appointment for activity or setting up some kind of contractual arrangement with your companions can mean the difference between doing it or not. I am fortunate in this respect. For years I have had the benefit of "personal trainers" who get me out for a 3-mile walk or jog at 6:30 *every* morning, and again for 2 miles at around 5:00 *every* afternoon. Right now they are a German shepherd and an Akita/shepherd crossbreed. This has been our routine from the day they were adopted and arrived in our household. It became an essential part of *their* lifestyle as well as mine, and they absolutely insist on getting out at the appointed times. The shepherd comes to grab my hand or my pant leg if I tend to be a bit tardy. So, if you can't find (or don't prefer) human companionship, visit your local Humane Society and adopt a pet. If you have some concerns about safety when you go out for a walk, get a big one!

In addition to whatever main approach you use to increase physical activity—5- or 10-minute periods, longer walks, or an active sport—there are a number of other things you can do that will add up to a good deal more movement during the day. When I was involved in daily work at the university I scheduled meetings and other appointments in other people's offices. Across campus, counting to and fro, it could total a mile or more of extra walking. In my own building, meeting in a colleague's office could add two flights of stairs each way and a quarter-mile walk. I continue to use stairs instead of elevators, at least for several flights, and in supermarket parking lots my car is usually the farthest from the door. I get an extra walk when I return the shopping cart to the store. Although I won't replace my computer and word processor for my old manual typewriter, I use manual can openers, hand beaters rather than electrical when I cook, and manual rather than electrical tools for home repairs whenever possible. Think about your own situation and replace a little of the electrical energy you are now using in your daily life with your own muscle. There's a real likelihood that you will be healthier as a result.

Dealing with Stress

There are several kinds of stresses in our lives. Those that are seen as challenges that we feel quite confident we can handle, even if they require great mental or physical effort, arouse and excite us and actually contribute to our vitality. When we face challenges of this kind, we usually find it easy to release tension and relax when we take a work break or when work is finished for the day.

But if there is an important area of your life—your work or a personal relationship—where the outcome is uncertain or your needs are not being met no matter how hard you seem to try, the associated stress can be a real danger to your health. Stress depresses the immune system, and while there is no firm evidence that it can play a part in the development of cancer, there is plenty of evidence linking it to an increased susceptibility to infection and hypertension. Under certain conditions, acute stress can bring on a heart attack. For example, a cardiologist told me about one of his patients who arrived home after a big evening meal and several alcoholic drinks to find the house ransacked and his most valued treasures stolen. He suffered a fatal heart attack on the spot. The physician thought the heavy meal and alcoholic drinks probably contributed to the deadly seriousness of the attack.

I'd like to give you some advice that can put you on the right path toward dealing with both chronic and acute stress. If the immediate steps I suggest don't result in your being able to deal adequately with the stresses in your life, go on and try my further recommendations.

IMMEDIATE STEPS

The first steps toward effectively dealing with stress lie entirely in your hands. Since saying them is a little easier than doing them, I'll give you some exact procedures to follow.

The best, if sometimes the most difficult, way to alleviate stress is to remove the cause at its source. Sometimes this is possible, realistically, and sometimes it's not. When it is, at work and in interpersonal relationships, it can mean talking it out with a boss, other colleagues, a mate or lover, or the relation or friend who plays a part in creating the stress. And remember, asserting your needs or feelings is different from being hostile. Simply saying "I feel such and such" when something occurs, and suggesting an alternative or some negotiations, is different from putting it in a way that blames the other person for your feelings and possibly antagonizes that person, for example, "YOU *make me feel* such and such."

When I had a private clinical practice, one of the books that I recommended to my clients who had trouble coping with other people in important situations was *When I Say No, I Feel Guilty*, by Manuel J. Smith, published by Bantam Books. Although written 20 years ago, this book retains its usefulness. You will find many others of its genre in the self-help section of your favorite bookstore. If a book of this kind doesn't help, there are three other levels of help you can and should look toward.

First, talking with a family member or friend who listens and helps you, yourself, design possible courses of action is your very first line of defense. However, many people with the best intentions have a way of offering suggestions that makes the other person even more tense than they were to begin with. You don't need to avoid such companionship, but you may find it more relaxing to be with such people if you don't discuss your problems!

Second, if a helpful family member or friend is not available or if talking with them doesn't help, you might discuss the issue with your minister, priest, or rabbi, or other religious leader, if they offer such counseling to members of their congregations.

Third, if that doesn't help, depending on the problem, find a professional management, psychological, family, or marital counselor with experience in dealing with your kind of problem. Be assured that the great majority of people who turn to professional help *do* report that it's helpful. If the first professional you turn to does not prove congenial, don't hesitate to try someone else. A comfortable personal relationship between client and counselor is important.

Sometimes there is no way to remove the source of stress in a person's life. Attempting to talk with a boss can really mean the loss of a job, and sometimes, in today's business world, you can find yourself without a job through no fault of your own as a company downsizes or merges with another. Here it can be a question of attitude, putting things in perspective, and digging into your own personal well of ingenuity and determination.

SPECIFIC SUGGESTIONS FOR DEALING WITH WORK STRESS

A majority of Americans report that being overburdened at work, or being dissatisfied with the kind of work they feel locked into, is the primary source of stress in their lives. About two-thirds of all workers do not look forward to their day's work, and, from CEOs and top-level managers to office workers, from 25 to 33 percent say they would choose a different career if they had it to do over again.

Since it's often impossible to remove work stress at its source, most people attempt to alleviate it by other means. Talking and joking with colleagues can be helpful, as can taking an exercise break or a walk at lunchtime. Physical activity is a great stress reducer, whether you choose the 5-minutes-per-hour routine, a walk early in the morning before work, or a visit to the gym afterward. In fact, when my wife was at her busiest teaching (as professor of music at Vanderbilt University) and at the same time practicing 4 hours a day while keeping up her concert career, she went to the YMCA after work to exercise and relax before coming home in order to achieve a mental state that would permit civil conversation.

Exercise is indeed one of the best stress reducers, along with the relaxation and meditation techniques described below. If chronic, unavoidable stress goes with the territory in your life, I strongly advise that you try to build in a 40-minute (or longer) walk in some pleasant environment at some point every day. Being alone in a pleasant spot, in physical movement, with time to reflect and plan, can be a refreshing and relaxing "mini-vacation" from your daily stresses.

And, if you watch any television at all, don't say you have no time for such activity. Watching TV does not reduce stress, and may, if you evaluate how you feel after watching, even be adding to a feeling of tension and a sense of unfulfillment in your life. Convert your TV time into something more profitable and healthful, beginning with physical activity. Or think about some other activity—it doesn't have to be physical—that might play a more rewarding part in your life.

What I am suggesting here can be especially helpful to you if your work is not rewarding. If there is a skill or hobby that you have always wanted to develop or pursue, give it a shot now. Something that you like to do and which gives you pleasure in your off-work hours will make your work feel less stressful and give you something to look forward to every day. Doing something pleasurable, or having something pleasurable to look forward to, is one of the most effective stress reducers.

There are, however, certain kinds of pleasurable stress-reducing strategies that I think you should avoid. Since eating, drinking, and smoking can reduce tension, people often find themselves trying to relax by consuming coffee, soft drinks, and unhealthful sweet, fatty snack foods or lighting up a cigarette during work breaks. Some have an alcoholic beverage or two at lunchtime to wind down. These approaches to stress reduction either serve to maintain the physiological tension or add to the risk of the degenerative diseases you are trying to avoid with the Cancer Prevention Good Health Diet. However, since having something to drink can help refresh you, I suggest you try hot or iced tea (use decaffeinated or herbal if regular is too stimulating) or iced plain or carbonated water, flavored if you like with bit of lemon or orange peel. Keep a cup or glass handy and take a sip frequently throughout the day.

MENTAL STRESS REDUCERS

Because doing or thinking about pleasurable things helps reduce stress, many people find it useful to take occasional "vision breaks" during the day. Two kinds of visions can be surprisingly helpful and I suggest you experiment a little with them.

When you feel tense, take a few minutes off and imagine you are in a favorite spot, or create a make-believe, pleasant scene of any kind in your mind, for example, lying on a beach or hillside on a warm summer's day. Just experience it—don't try to do anything; simply keep it in your mind's eye. Or, as a second kind of vision, think about something pleasant that you like to do or plan to do later in the day or week. If you play tennis or golf, mentally practice some aspect of your sport—your serve, forehand, drive, or putt. Or, if you like to walk or jog, take a mental walk or jog in your favorite environment for a few minutes if you can't actually get up and do it.

I have included in Appendix B instructions for how to perform two of the most effective stress reducers I know of: deep muscular relaxation and meditation.

The deep muscular relaxation exercise will show you how to achieve almost instant physical and mental relaxation with a deep-breathing technique used by athletes when they need to calm themselves at critical times. You may have seen basketball players use it before shooting their foul shots. Racing biathalon skiers practice it and use it to reduce their heart rates by as much as 30 percent or more when they drop to the ground before firing at their targets. With as little as one or two days of practice you can learn to achieve an instant physiological effect, including, to begin with, about a 10 percent reduction in heart rate, as well as immediate relaxation in the parts of your body where tension accumulates, such as around your shoulders and neck. Try it out, and if it appeals to you, you will get even better with more practice. Once learned, many people find that the relaxation response becomes their automatic reaction to stressful situations, and actually short-circuits the stress experience.

The meditational approach that I suggest in Appendix B has proven to be helpful in the control of hypertension as well as in the reduction of stress.

Reducing the Dangers to Your Health in Your Home and Work Environments

MAINTAINING A HEALTHFUL HOME ENVIRONMENT

Experts estimate that only about 2 percent of all cancer deaths are related to environmental pollution, but any one of a number of pollutants can play a significant role in any individual case, and often a greater role in heart disease and other diseases than in cancer.

For example, while secondhand smoke may play a significant role in the deaths of "only" about 4000 people each year from lung cancer, in actuality this type of environmental pollution contributes to about 50,000 deaths each year, of which about 35,000 are from heart disease. And living with a smoker or working in a smoke-filled environment can increase your risk of cancer, heart disease, respiratory infections, or asthma from 30 to 200 percent.

The risk of secondhand smoke played a key role in my own decision not to continue smoking cigars, which I very much enjoyed. When I began working with computers in 1983 I carefully avoided lighting up a cigar in my computer room since the smoke contained many contaminants that could guck up the computer and cause it to malfunction.[1] I would go out to the study, where my wife might be reading, and light up. One day, when she started to cough, it suddenly became obvious to me that I was doing something pretty stupid—guarding my computer so carefully while endangering the life of my wife as well as my own. That one thought was enough—I have never since smoked another cigar.

In addition to secondhand tobacco smoke, radon, asbestos, pesticides, household cleaners and other products, drinking water, and electromagnetic fields may pose some increased risk for cancer in the home.

Radon. Radon is a radioactive gas released in soil, water, and rocks as uranium breaks down in the earth. The Environmental Protection Agency (EPA) estimates that several million homes in the United States have dangerous levels of radon seeping in from the earth through cracks in their foundations and walls. Radon testing kits that meet EPA testing requirements are available from most hardware stores for around $25 to $30. You can obtain more information about how to protect yourself and your fam-

---

[1]If you are a smoker, or work in an area permeated by tobacco smoke, take a look at any glass or mirrored surface and you will see the film deposited by the particles in tobacco smoke.

ily from radon by writing or calling the U.S. Environmental Protection Agency Information Access Branch, Public Information Center, 401 M Street, S.W., Washington, D.C. 20460 (202-260-2080).

Asbestos. Once popular as a building and insulating material, asbestos only becomes dangerous when it is damaged and microscopic particles are released to float in the air where they can be inhaled, lodge in the lungs, and seriously increase the risk of cancer. If you live in an older home or work in an older building, especially those built before 1950, there is some likelihood that insulation, floor tiles, patching compounds, and other building materials contain asbestos. If these materials are in good shape, there is little to worry about and they should not be disturbed except by experts who know how to handle the material correctly. For more information on how to deal with asbestos you can contact the Toxic Substance Control Act Administration Office, 401 M Street, S.W., Washington, D.C. 20460 (202-554-1404).

Pesticides and Cleaning Fluids. Pesticides are a special danger to children and pets. They should be used in the smallest amounts that can get the job done, whether inside the home or outside, on lawns and gardens. When and if the use of a pesticide is necessary and you plan to apply it yourself, read the label and follow the instructions carefully. This is also important when you use cleaning fluids and solvents in your home, especially liquid paint strippers, paints, and lubricants. According to the EPA, most commercial pesticide services appear to be reliable and they should be able to answer any of your questions about the chemicals they are using. However, I have been informed of two instances locally in which birds and small animals died in the vicinity of lawns that had recently been chemically treated, and my own experience with the pesticide firm that had been treating the house we now live in for the previous owners, on a monthly basis, was not good. We retained the firm, but found that they greatly overdosed the place. We could not stand to stay in the house for the rest of the day after each visit. We discharged the firm after the second month. For more information before employing a commercial service, you can contact the National Pesticide Telecommunications Network at 800-858-7378 for advice on various chemicals and guidelines for their application.

Drinking Water. There have been numerous recent reports questioning the safety of drinking water in many parts of the country. Although the major concern is with certain infectious diseases, there is also some debate about organic compounds that combine with chlorine and may have some carcinogenic activity. The EPA maintains a Safe Drinking Water Hotline (800-426-4791) to answer questions about water safety, and municipal water services will send you a report on the local supply on request. If you obtain your water from a well, you should have it tested (testing companies are listed in the Yellow Pages of your phone book under a "water" heading, such as "Water Analysis" or "Water Treatment"). I recommend that everyone use a home water filter that removes organic compounds and chlorine because, first, it makes water taste good and clean again, the way it should. Most people don't drink enough plain water because it smells and tastes bad directly from the faucet. In addition to improving the taste of water itself, filtering will greatly improve the taste of tea, coffee, and other beverages. Unless your water is dangerously high in certain metals or minerals, I don't recommend the kind of water filter that removes these in addition to organic compounds because water is often a source of important minerals, such as calcium and magnesium.

Electromagnetic Fields. Some reports suggest that electromagnetic fields can increase the risk of certain cancers, especially leukemia in children. But unless you are willing to live miles away from any electricity, you cannot completely avoid them. All electrical appliances generate electromagnetic fields, however slight, and no one really knows if an absolutely safe level exists. Since the strength of the field diminishes very rapidly with distance, the best advice is to simply place your body as far from an electrical gadget as possible when it is operating, including your monitor if you work with a computer. While it's also easy to distance yourself from other appliances, such as your toaster or microwave (and a down comforter and flannel sheets are excellent replacements for an electric blanket), it's hardly possible to place your body far away from an electric shaver or hair dryer and still use them for their intended purposes. So here's yet another reason to substitute the manual for the electrical whenever possible. If you have any concerns about electromagnetic fields in your home, you can call your electric company for an evaluation. Most companies have a person who will do this free of charge, and this person may be able to give you some advice if any appliance or area of your home has an unusually strong field.

X-RAYS

Normally the danger from X-rays is minimal, but most experts suggest that you avoid them whenever it is prudent. For example, always ask your doctor and dentist the reason for an X-ray if a compelling one is not immediately evident to you, and make sure you avoid duplication if you use the services of different doctors. I use two different dentists, and, unless I force them to consult with each other, they will each order their own set of X-rays periodically. That's unnecessary, of course, since one can report to the other the latest results.

CARCINOGENS IN THE WORKPLACE

The list of chemicals and other agents that are known or potential carcinogens in many occupations is distressingly long. It numbers in the thousands. *If you work for a manufacturer of metal products or around any kind of chemical solvent, petroleum product, dye, dust, smoke, or radioactive material, your employer should inform you of known dangers.* You may also consult the U.S. Department of Labor's Occupational Safety and Health Administration (OSHA) for information about your particular situation. If you feel you are being exposed unnecessarily, you can also obtain information on how to file a complaint: contact OSHA at 200 Constitution Avenue, N.W., Washington, D.C. 20210 (202-219-9308); you may be referred to a regional office closer to you.

Unfortunately, OSHA-permissible exposure limits to many substances may be outdated and inaccurate. You cannot assume you are safe just because your situation meets government-permissible levels. You, yourself, must do everything you can to protect yourself. Follow all safety procedures, wear the correct protective clothing for your job, and wash, clean, and/or vacuum yourself and your work clothing if you work in an industry that exposes you to known or possible carcinogens. Whatever you do, if you are a smoker, QUIT. Tobacco smoke greatly enhances the impact of many other carcinogenic substances, increasing your risk in certain cases from 2 to as much as 15 times the risk of each substance alone.

A ONE-STOP RESOURCE FOR FURTHER INFORMATION AND ADVICE ON HOW TO DEAL WITH CANCER-RELATED HEALTH HAZARDS IN YOUR HOME AND WORKPLACE

The American Cancer Society maintains a Cancer Answer Line accessible through 800-227-2345. When you dial this number from any place in the United States, your call is directed to your state office, where a person is available to answer your questions.

Epilogue

I have tried in this book to do more than just tell you *what* to do to double the likelihood of adding up to 20 or more years to your "health span." I've tried to show you *how* to do it in simple steps: first, by experimenting with two or three new plant-based recipes each week, and then, as you find dishes you like, designing more and more of your meals centered on plant foods. I've tried to show you that good health can taste good too, by illustrating, in my recipes, ways to make vegetables, fruits, and grains so tasty and satisfying that you will find it easy to cut back on the most dangerous items in the average American diet: too much fat (especially saturated fat), too many calories, and too much red meat. If you follow my suggestions, I think you will find yourself eating a much more nutritious diet in a matter of a few weeks or months, and the change will have taken place with little effort and no deprivation.

The most important Cancer Prevention Good Health guidelines include eating a wide variety of different fruits and vegetables so that you cover all the bases and include the many different phytochemicals that can bolster your immune system and block or suppress the development of various degenerative diseases before they can obtain a foothold in your body. Color is one key: By including at least three different colors of fruits and vegetables in your diet each day—for example, red, yellow/orange, and green—you obtain a number of different phytochemicals with preventive powers. But all colors can represent important phytochemicals and the more variety you include in your meal plans, the better!

There is, of course, more to it than color alone. Different families of plant foods are just as important, including cruciferous vegetables; onion, garlic, and related foods; beans, particularly soybeans and soy products; and various fruits, especially citrus fruit.

If you are a sedentary person I hope I have convinced you to use one of my strategies for becoming more active. Even if you can't find a way to move about briskly in a single 45- to 60-minute period almost every day, just getting up and out of your chair for 5 minutes on the hour during waking hours can make a real difference in weight management and stress reduction. And, if you move around energetically, it can increase fitness and contribute to reducing your risk of virtually all degenerative illnesses.

We are all exposed to carcinogenic substances every day. They are all around us and some are simply unavoidable. Your first line of defense lies in your diet. By following the guidelines I have laid out in this book, you can cut your risk at least in half.

But before concluding, I must issue a word of warning.

As might be expected, those who package supplements have begun touting pills that supposedly contain the disease-fighting phytochemicals I've been talking about. One advertisement that I have just received makes only a modest claim for one of its supplements—that it contains the amount of a single anticarcinogenic isothiocyanate, sulphoraphane, equal to 2 servings of broccoli. But another advertisement claims its supplement to be equal to 25 pounds of broccoli!

BE WARNED! While you have in reality no assurance that supplements contain what their manufacturers and marketing agents claim is in them (and laboratory tests show they frequently don't), even if they do, any phytochemical, taken singly in excessive quantities, *may be extremely dangerous.* The very substance that blocks or suppresses the development of cancer as found naturally in foods, where it occurs balanced with hundreds of other phytochemicals *that work together,* CAN BECOME CARCINOGENIC WHEN CONSUMED SINGLY IN LARGE DOSES. It may take a few years, but a supplement that contains any phytochemical equal to the amount found in 25 pounds of any food may end up killing you, rather than contributing to your health and well-being.

So, let's stick with the facts: people who eat the most plant foods have half (or less) the risk of developing cancer and heart disease compared with people who eat the least. I've tried to show you how to bring your own diet into line with these findings, and I want to wish you a long, happy, and healthy life.

. . .

If you have any problems following my advice you may write to me and I will do my best to be helpful. I do answer my mail, although sometimes, if I'm traveling, it may take a few weeks. Please do not call on the telephone since the volume of calls is often more than I can handle. Of course, I am always happy to hear of your success, especially how you deal with problems along the way, and, in my lectures, as an inspiration to others, I often quote from letters that I have received.

Please address your correspondence to:

Martin Katahn
4607 Belmont Park Terrace
Nashville, TN 37215

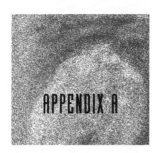

The Scientific Background: Selected Bibliography

I located over 1200 research articles and consulted a number of general references in order to gather information on the relationship of diet and other components of a person's lifestyle to the development of cancer, cardiovascular disease, and other degenerative diseases. Those that I consider most important and most likely to be useful to my readers are listed here, with annotations when the titles do not adequately convey the nature of the contents. Part 1 lists texts, books, and encyclopedias; Part 2, health-oriented newsletters; and Part 3, key research studies, reviews, and theoretical articles.

Part 1

Baker, C. G., and Scarpelli, D. G. "Cancer." In *The New Encyclopaedia Britannica,* Vol. 15, pp. 555–64. Chicago: Encyclopaedia Britannica, Inc., 1989.

The most thorough and technical of the encyclopedic references that I consulted, this article discusses the origin, developmental progression, types, and treatment of various cancers. I also made particular use of information obtained from the article on cancer by Charles Mason Huguley, Jr., in the multimedia encyclopedia *Microsoft Encarta '95.* I found other helpful encyclopedia articles on cancer in *Compton's Interactive Encyclopedia, Edition 1995* (by Serena Stockwell), and in *The 1995 Grolier Multimedia Encyclopedia* (by Henry C. Pitot).

Harborne, J. B. *Introduction to Ecological Biochemistry.* San Diego: Academic Press, 1993.

A text in phytochemical ecology, this book describes how plant biochemistry evolved through plants' interactions with animal and other environmental influences and provides information on the chemical structures of different plants, as well as the distribution and physiological activity of these structures.

Herbert, V., and Subak-Sharpe, G. J., eds. *Total Nutrition: The Only Guide You'll Ever Need.* New York: St. Martin's Press, 1995.

Arguments against vitamin and mineral supplementation are presented in Chapter 1, "What Is a Healthy Food Plan?," by Victor Herbert and Tracy Stopler Kasdan, pp. 3–16, and Chapter 7, "Vitamins and Minerals Plus Antioxidant Supplements," by Victor Herbert, pp. 94–118.

Messina, M., and Messina, V. K. "Vegetables: Rating the Healthiest." In *Encyclopaedia Britannica: Medical and Health Annual,* pp. 289–94. Chicago: Encyclopaedia Britannica, Inc., 1996.

The *Medical and Health Annuals* of the Encyclopaedia Britannica present summaries of the latest research in the field, including the relationship of diet to disease. This article in particular, under the subhead "A Close Look at Phytochemicals" (pp. 290–91), discusses the special health benefits of a variety of vegetables and other plant foods.

Shils, M. E., Olson, J. A., and Shike, M., eds. *Modern Nutrition in Health and Disease.* Philadelphia: Lea & Febiger, 1994.

This is an exhaustive technical reference; scientific background information in *The Cancer Prevention Good Health Diet* was drawn from the following chapters: "Oxidative Stress, Oxidant Defense, and Dietary Constituents," by James A. Thomas (Chapter 33, pp. 501–12); "Fads, Frauds, and Quackery," by Stephen Barrett and Victor Herbert (Chapter 86, pp. 1526–32); "Cardiovascular Disease," by Donald J. McNamara (Chapter 87, pp. 1533–44); and "Diet, Cancer, and Food Safety," by Michael W. Pariza (Chapter 88, pp. 1545–58).

Tyler, V. E. *The Honest Herbal: A Sensible Guide to the Use of Herbs and Related Remedies.* New York: Pharmaceutical Products Press, 1993.

This book provides information on the chemical structure and physiological activity of herbs and related remedies, with assessment of effectiveness and safety, arranged alphabetically by common plant name.

Tyler, V. E. *Herbs of Choice: The Therapeutic Use of Phytomedicinals.* New York: Pharmaceutical Products Press, 1994.

This book describes the therapeutic use of phytomedicinals as preventives and remedies for various physical ailments, arranged according to problem areas. I drew information from "Cardiovascular System Problems" (pp. 101–15) and "Cancer" (pp. 177–81).

Webb, D., and Smith, S. M. *Food for Better Health.* Lincolnwood, Ill.: Publications International, Ltd., 1995.

The authors present basic information on essential nutrients and the relationship of diet to various diseases, with information about and recipes for their Top 100 foods.

Whitney, E. N., Cataldo, C. B., and Rolfes, S. R. *Understanding Normal and Clinical Nutrition*. Minneapolis/St. Paul: West Publishing Company, 1994.

This is a comprehensive college text that I use as my primary reference in the field of nutrition. Appendix B provides the background in chemistry that's needed to understand nutrition concepts. The discussion of chemical reactions and the formation of free radicals in this appendix is especially useful in understanding the carcinogenic process.

Winawer, S. J., and Shike, M. *Cancer Free*. New York: Simon & Schuster, 1995.

This valuable book includes advice on how to assess your personal risk for various cancers; prevention, screening, and treatment, with exhaustive lists of environmental and genetic factors involved; and sources of further information and advice for dealing with every form of this disease.

Part 2

The following representative articles from a number of reputable newsletters in the health area contain supplemental information on many of the topics covered in *The Cancer Prevention Good Health Diet*. The articles are based on the latest research appearing in respected, peer-reviewed scientific journals. They are written with a minimum of technical jargon and in a style that makes the information easy to understand and put into practice.

"Can Aspirin Protect You from Cancer?," *University of California at Berkeley Wellness Letter,* December 1995.

"Cancer: What You Eat Can Affect Your Risk," *Mayo Clinic Health Letter,* September 1995.

"Colon Cancer: Diet May Hold Key to Prevention of This Common Killer," *Environmental Nutrition,* April 1995.

"Dodging Cancer with Diet," *Nutrition Action Healthletter,* January/February 1995 (article by Bonnie Liebman).

"Does Exercise Build Immunity?," *Consumer Reports on Health,* April 1995.

"Does Stress Kill?," *Consumer Reports on Health,* July 1995.

"Eating More Fat Means Storing More Fat," *Running and FitNews,* November 1995 (a summary of a study appearing in the *American Journal of Clinical Nutrition,* 1995, Vol. 62, No. 1, pp. 19–29, as this book went to press, which "clearly reinforces the importance of dietary fat as the primary factor in weight management"; it further notes that "more total fat is stored when the excess [overfeeding] is fat compared with carbohydrate").

"Fiber Bounces Back," *Consumer Reports on Health,* March 1995.

"Green Revolution," *Harvard Health Letter: Special Supplement,* April 1995 (on phytochemical properties of cancer-fighting foods).

"Is Our Water Safety Going Down the Drain?," *University of California at Berkeley Wellness Letter,* September 1995.

"Lung and Prostate Cancers Are Top Killers: Can Diet Help?," *Environmental Nutrition,* September 1995.

"Melatonin: Sleep Aid, Jet-Lag Antidote, Plus the Promise of Much More," *Environmental Nutrition,* November 1995.

"More than a Hill of Beans: Soy Research Takes Off," *American Institute for Cancer Research Newsletter,* Fall 1995.

"Reading Tea Leaves for Health Benefits," *Tufts University Diet & Nutrition Letter: Special Report,* October 1995 (evidence for the beneficial effects of tea in the prevention of cancer and heart disease).

"Respect Grows for Botanicals, but Can You Trust the Herbs You Buy?," *Environmental Nutrition,* May 1995.

"Take Time for Teatime," *American Institute for Cancer Research Newsletter,* Fall 1995.

"Those Mighty Phytochemicals: Beyond the Benefits of Broccoli," *Environmental Nutrition,* November 1995.

Part 3

The following is a selection of representative recent research and review articles that provide information relating dietary specifics to some aspect of cancer, and in some cases to other degenerative diseases, as will be noted in the title or annotations. The individual research articles listed are not one-shot deals; they represent recent findings in an ongoing line of research. By examining the article listed here and its references, a reader interested in that particular research topic will be able to pursue the area in depth.

Adlercreutz, H., and Mazur, W., "Phyto-oestrogens and Western Diseases," *Annals of Medicine,* 29, No. 2 (1997):95–120.

Isoflavonoids (found in legumes) and lignans (found in many different plant fibers) may play a significant inhibitory role in cancer development, particularly in the promotional phase of the disease. Recent evidence suggests that they may also play a preventive role in the initiation stage of carcinogenesis.

Ames, B. N., Shigenaga, M. K., and Gold, L. S., "DNA Lesions, Inducible DNA Repair, and Cell Division: Three Key Factors in Mutagenesis and Carcinogenesis," *Environmental Health Perspectives*, 101, Suppl. 5 (1993):35–44.

This article describes various events within the cell that can damage it and result in cancer, together with the systems of defenses that work to repair the damage and prevent the progression of the disease. It also describes how exogenous agents (for example, phytochemicals in food) can increase the effectiveness of the defenses.

Azuine, M. A., and Bhide, S. V., "Adjuvant Chemoprevention of Experimental Cancer: Catechin and Dietary Turmeric in Forestomach and Oral Cancer Models," *Journal of Ethnopharmacology*, 44, No. 3 (1994):211–17.

Catechin and turmeric, which are commonly consumed natural products, showed effective chemopreventive activity in mice and golden hamsters.

Bairati, I., Meyer, F., Fradet, Y., and Moore, L., "Dietary Fat and Advanced Prostate Cancer," *Journal of Urology*, 159, No. 4 (1998):1271–75.

A high intake of saturated fat and total fat from animal sources appears to encourage the progression of prostate cancer.

Barch, D. H., Rundhaugen, L. M., and Pillay, N. S., "Ellagic Acid Induces Transcription of the Rat Glutathione S-Transferase-YA Gene," *Carcinogenesis*, 16, No. 3 (1995):665–68.

Ellagic acid facilitated the production of glutathione S-transferase enzymes, the enzymes that detoxify carcinogens and prevent or reduce mutations that lead to the growth of tumors.

Chen, X. G., and Han, R., ["Effect of Glycyrrhetinic Acid on DNA Damage and Unscheduled DNA Synthesis Induced by Benzo[a]pyrene"], *Yao Hsueh Hsueh Pao* [*Acta Pharmaceutica Sinica*], 29, No. 10 (1994):725–29. (Published in Chinese, English summary from Medline.)

Glycyrrhetinic acid (found in licorice) at calculated doses had both a blocking and suppressing impact when administered to experimental animals subjected to known carcinogenic agents. The authors concluded by suggesting that "glycyrrhetinic acid has effective anti-initiating and anti-promoting activities and could be used for cancer chemopreventive purpose."

Colditz, G. A., Cannuscio, C. C., and Frazier, A. L., "Physical Activity and Reduced Risk of Colon Cancer: Implications for Prevention," *Cancer Causes and Control*, 8, No. 4, (1997):649–67.

A high level of physical activity, either occupational or recreational, was associated with a 50 percent reduction in the risk of colon cancer.

Dashwood, R. H., "Early Detection and Prevention of Colorectal Cancer (Review)," *Oncology Reports*, No. 2 (1999):277–81.

Many different phytochemicals have been identified as potential inhibitors of colorectal cancer, but no single one can be recommended for wide-scale use in humans at this time for lack of information on mechanisms of action. From his review of the literature, the author concludes that the best approach to reducing the risk of colorectal cancer would be to increase the dietary intake of fruits, vegetables, and cereals, and to reduce the intake of fat, particularly from animal sources.

Decker, E. A., "The Role of Phenolics, Conjugated Linoleic Acid, Carnosine, and Pyrroloquinoline Quinone as Nonessential Dietary Antioxidants," *Nutrition Reviews*, 53, No. 3 (1995):49–58.

This review describes the role of the body's own antioxidant systems and examines the potential of various phytochemicals that inhibit oxidative reactions in food and biological tissues.

De Stefani, E., Fontham, E. T., Chen, V., Correa, P., Deneo-Pellegrini, H., Ronco, A., and Mendilaharsu, M., "Fatty Foods and the Risk of Lung Cancer: A Case-control Study from Uruguay," *International Journal of Cancer*, 71, No. 5 (1997):760–66.

Both fat-rich and sucrose-rich foods were associated with an increased risk of lung cancer.

Dragsted, L. O., Strube, M., and Larsen, J. C., "Cancer-Protective Factors in Fruits and Vegetables: Biochemical and Biological Background," *Pharmacology and Toxicology*, 72S (1993):116–34.

A key review article summarizing evidence for the mechanisms of action of cancer-protective agents in fruits and vegetables. The material on blocking and suppressing the progression of cancer in Chapter 3 of *The Cancer Prevention Good Health Diet* is drawn to a great extent from this article.

Franceschi, S., Parpinel, M., La Vecchia, C., Favero, A., Talamini, R., and Negri, E., "Role of Different Types of Vegetables and Fruit in the Prevention of Cancer of the Colon, Rectum, and Breast," *Epidemiology*, 9, No. 3 (1998):338–41.

Looking at thousands of different cancer cases and comparing them with controls (patients who did not suffer from any form of cancer) the authors found that consumption of most vegetables reduced the risk of cancer of the colon and rectum. Only carrots and vegetables consumed raw were associated with reduced risk of breast cancer, while high fruit consumption was specifically related to a reduced incidence of rectal cancer.

Franke, A. A., Mordan, L. J., Cooney, R. V., Harwood, P. J., and Wang, W., "Dietary Phenolic Agents Inhibit Neoplastic Transformation and Trap Toxic NO_2," (meeting abstract), *Proceedings of the Annual Meeting of the American Association for Cancer Research*, 36 (1995):A741.

Most of the phenols examined proved to be equal to or superior to carotenoids and vitamins in their inhibitory effects.

Goodman, M. T., Hankin, J. H., Wilkens, L. R., Lyu, L., McDuffie, K., Liu, L. Q., and Kolonel, L. N., "Diet, Body Size, Physical Activity, and the Risk of Endometrial Cancer," *Cancer Research,* 57, No. 22 (1997):5077–85.

A high-fat diet was associated with an increased risk of endometrial cancer in obese women, while a diet rich in plant foods was associated with a reduced risk.

Greenwald, P., Kelloff, G., Burch-Whitman, C., and Kramer, B. S., "Chemoprevention," *CA A Cancer Journal for Clinicians,* 45 (1995):31–49.

A review of theory, research, and programs in the area of chemoprevention, with emphasis on the future importance of the chemoprevention of cancer.

Hankin, J. H., "Role of Nutrition in Women's Health: Diet and Breast Cancer," *Journal of the American Dietetic Association,* 93, No. 9 (1993):994–999.

An analysis of 12 different case-control studies showed a 50 percent increase in the relative risk for breast cancer among postmenopausal women with high intakes of saturated fat. This adds support to the findings of a causal relationship reported in animal research and international correlational studies. The author suggests that inconsistencies among research studies may be due to the difficulty of collecting accurate dietary information and other methodological limitations.

Hecht, S. S., Staretz, M. E., Yang, C. S., Smith, T. J., Stoner, G. D., Morse, M. A., Smith, C. E., Jiao, D., and Chung, F. L., "Isothiocyanates: Novel Chemopreventive Agents for Lung Cancer" (meeting abstract), *Proceedings of the Annual Meeting of the American Association for Cancer Research,* 35 (1994):695–96.

Isothiocyanates (found in cruciferous vegetables and watercress) inhibited the metabolic activation and carcinogenicity in rat and mouse tissues of two of the most likely carcinogens in tobacco smoke, benzo[a]pyrene and a tobacco-specific nitrosamine.

Hirohata, T., and Kono, S., "Diet/Nutrition and Stomach Cancer in Japan," *International Journal of Cancer,* Suppl. 10:34–36.

Comparing Japanese living in their homeland with those living in Hawaii, the authors found that consumption of salt and salty foods is associated with an increased risk of stomach cancer, while consumption of vegetables and fruit is associated with reduced risk. The authors conclude by saying that the incidence of stomach cancer in Japan might be reduced by two-thirds via dietary changes such as have occurred in the Japanese now living in Hawaii.

Hsing, A. W., McLaughlin, J. K., Chow, W. H., Schuman, L. M., Co Chien, H. T., Gridley, G., Bjelke, E., Wacholder, S., and Blot, W. J., "Risk Factors for Colorectal Cancer in a Prospective Study among U.S. White Men," *International Journal of Cancer,* 77, No. 4 (1998):549–53.

Looking at a 20-year follow-up in a group of over 17,000 men, the authors found that a high intake of red meat and a sedentary lifestyle almost doubled the risk of colon cancer.

Izzotti, A., De Flora, S., Petrilli, G. L., Gallagher, J., Rojas, M., Alexandrov, K., Bartsch, H., and Lewtas, J., "Cancer Biomarkers in Human Atherosclerotic Lesions: Detection of DNA Adducts," *Cancer Epidemiology, Biomarkers and Prevention* 4, No. 2 (1995):105–10.

Looking at changes in the DNA in atherosclerotic lesions in the aorta, the authors concluded that their data provided further support for the hypothesis that "there may be similarities between the carcinogenic and the atherogenic processes, and in particular that genetic alterations caused by DNA-binding agents in the artery wall may be detected in atherosclerotic lesions."

Jones, L. A., Gonzalez, R., Pillow, P. C., Gomez-Garza, S. A., Foreman, C. J., Chilton, J. A., Linares, A., Yick, J., Badrei, M., and Hajek, R. A., "Dietary Fiber, Hispanics, and Breast Cancer Risk?" *Annals of the New York Academy of Sciences,* 837 (1997):524–36.

The low incidence of breast cancer in Hispanic women living in most regions of the United States may be related to the high intake of fiber in their diets.

Kim, I., Williamson, D. F., Byers, T., and Koplan, J. P., "Vitamin and Mineral Supplement Use and Mortality in a US Cohort," *American Journal of Public Health,* 83, No. 4 (1993):546–50.

Among a group of 10,758 studied, 22.5 percent took supplements daily and 10 percent took them at least once a week. No evidence was found for increased longevity among users of vitamin and mineral supplements in the United States.

Koo, L. C., Mang, O. W., and Ho, J. H. C., "An Ecological Study of Trends in Cancer Incidence and Dietary Changes in Hong Kong," *Nutrition and Cancer,* 28, No. 3 (1997):289–301.

Looking at changes in diet and the incidence of various cancers that have occurred in the last 30 years in Hong Kong, the authors found that the increased intake of meat and its associated fat are related to the increase in colon, rectal, prostate, and breast cancers.

Kushi, L. H., Potter, J. D., Bostick, R. M., Drinkard, C. R., Sellers, T. A., Gapstur, S. M., Cerhan, J. R., and Folsom, A. R., "Dietary Fat and Risk of Breast Cancer According to Hormone Receptor Status," *Cancer Epidemiology, Biomarkers and Prevention,* 4, No. 1 (1995):11–19.

The results of this study suggest that dietary fat may be an important risk factor for breast cancer only when both estrogen and progesterone hormone receptors are active in tissue. There may be no risk if either kind of receptor is inactive. Failure to control for type of receptor activity in different studies may help explain inconsistent results relating dietary fat to the risk of breast cancer.

Lee, I. M., "Antioxidant Vitamins in the Prevention of Cancer." *Proceedings of the Association of American Physicians,* 111, No. 1 (1999):10–15.

When individual antioxidant vitamins are examined in various kinds of studies (observational vs. more tightly controlled experimental studies) the evidence in support of individual nutrients as cancer prevention agents is inconsistent and controversial. The author concludes that available evidence suggests the risk of developing cancer is best reduced by the consumption of a diet rich in fruits and vegetables rather than in the consumption of specific antioxidant vitamin supplements.

Lee, M. M., Wang, R. T., Hsing, A. W., Gu, F. L., Wang, T., and Spitz, M., "Case-control Study of Diet and Prostate Cancer in China," *Cancer Causes and Control,* 9, No. 6 (1998):545–52.

The incidence of prostate cancer is much higher among men in the Western world than it is in China, and a high fat intake in the Western world is thought to be one of the risk factors. This study looked at native Chinese and found that even in a population with a generally low risk of prostate cancer, those men who suffered from the disease consumed significantly more fat than men in a comparison group living in similar neighborhoods who did not have the disease.

Leiss, J. K., and Savitz, D. A., "Home Pesticide Use and Childhood Cancer: A Case Control Study," *American Journal of Public Health,* 85, No. 2 (1995):249–52.

The authors found a greater incidence of certain cancers in children who grew up in homes subject to pesticide treatments of yards and use of pest strips.

Levi, F., Pasche, C., La Vecchia, C., Lucchini, F., and Franceschi, S., "Food Groups and Colorectal Cancer Risk." *British Journal of Cancer,* 79, Nos. 7–8 (1999):1283–87.

This study compared the diets of several hundred cancer patients with controls and found that a diet rich in refined grains and red meat increased the risk of colorectal cancer. The authors recommend that, to reduce the risk of colorectal cancer, whole grains be substituted for refined grains, intake of red meat reduced, and fruit and vegetable consumption increased.

Mayne, S. T., Janerich, D. T., Greenwald, P., Chorost, S., Tucci, C., Zaman, M. B., Melamed, M. R., Kiely, M., and McKneally, M. F., "Dietary Beta Carotene and Lung Cancer Risk in U.S. Nonsmokers," *Journal of the National Cancer Institute,* 86, No. 1 (1994):33–38.

The results of this case-control study suggested that dietary beta-carotene, raw fruits and vegetables, and vitamin E supplements can reduce the risk of lung cancer in non-smoking men and women.

Meyer, F., and White, E., "Alcohol and Nutrients in Relation to Colon Cancer in Middle-Aged Adults," *American Journal of Epidemiology,* 138, No. 4 (1993):225–36.

Alcohol consumption was found to be strongly related to an increased risk for colon cancer, while intake of dietary fiber was related to a lower relative risk.

Nijhoff, W. A., Bosboom, M. A., Smidt, M. H., and Peters, W. H., "Enhancement of Rat Hepatic and Gastrointestinal Glutathione and Glutathione S-Transferases by Alpha-Angelicalactone and Flavone," *Carcinogenesis,* 16, No. 3 (1995):607–12.

Naturally occurring anticarcinogens flavone and alpha-angelicalactone, when added in small amounts to the diet of animals, enhanced production of glutathione S-transferase enzymes in the liver and various areas of the gastrointestinal system, suggesting that chemopreventive effects can be obtained when these anticarcinogens are present at very low concentrations in the diet.

Ocké, M. C., Bueno-de-Mesquita, H. B., Feskens, E. J. M., van Staveren, W. A., and Kromhout, D., "Repeated Measurements of Vegetables, Fruits, Beta-carotene, and Vitamins C and E in Relation to Lung Cancer. The Zutphen Study," *American Journal of Epidemiology,* 145, No. 4 (1997):358–65.

The dietary habits and incidence of cancer in a group of 561 men were examined over a period of 30 years. Men with a high stable intake of fruits and vegetables during the period had less than half the risk of developing lung cancer than those with a low stable intake. Only beta-carotene, inferred from diet reports, had a significant beneficial impact.

Offord, E. A., Mace, K., Ruffieux, C., Aeschbach, R., Malnoe, A., and Pfeifer, A. M., "Mechanisms of Chemoprevention by Rosemary Antioxidants Studied in a Human Bronchial Epithelial Cell Model" (meeting abstract), *Proceedings of the Annual Meeting of the American Association for Cancer Research,* 36 (1995):A733.

Diterpenes found in rosemary have antioxidant and other chemopreventive properties; in this study they interfered with the action of a common carcinogen, preventing damage to DNA, while at the same time stimulating the production of protective enzymes.

Persky, V., "Soy and Cancer Risk: Epidemiologic Studies" (meeting abstract), *First International Symposium on the Role of Soy in Preventing and Treating Chronic Disease,* February 20–23, 1994, Mesa, Arizona, p. 11.

Studies have shown significant protection against breast, colon, lung, and stomach cancer for soy products (unfermented—not miso, but soy milk and tofu), with possible mechanisms of action being reduction of estrogen binding to receptors, inhibition of tyrosine protein kinases, induction of cytochrome P-450s and inhibition of DNA topoisomerases, and reduced methionine or increased protease inhibitors.

Potter, J. D., "Diet, Phytochemicals and Cancer Risk" (meeting abstract), *First International Symposium on the Role of Soy in Preventing and Treating Chronic Disease,* February 20–23, 1994, Mesa, Arizona, p. 10.

Includes lists of foods and phytochemicals that are believed to have healing and anticarcinogenic properties. "Vegetables and fruit contain the anticarcinogenic cocktail to which we are adapted. We abandon it at our peril."

Potter, J. D., and Steinmetz, K. A., "There Is More to Vegetables and Fruit than Antioxidants and Fiber," *Proceedings of the Annual Meeting of the American Association for Cancer Research,* 35 (1994):673–74.

This report summarizes evidence from epidemiological, cohort, and case-control studies linking specific plant foods, groups of plant foods, and various phytochemicals to the prevention of different kinds of cancers. "High consumption of vegetables and fruit means high intake of a wide variety of substances that keep enzyme systems 'tuned' to handle occasional high intakes of carcinogens; that act as substrates for endogenous production of anticarcinogens; that reduce the likelihood of damage to DNA; and that reduce the capacity of transformed cells to proliferate."

Rao, A. R., and Hashim, S., "Chemopreventive Action of Oriental Food-Seasoning Spice Mixture Garam Masala on DMBA-Induced Transplacental and Translactational Carcinogenesis in Mice," *Nutrition and Cancer,* 23, No. 1 (1995):91–101.

Small doses (10 and 30 milligrams) of garam masala resulted in significant reduction in tumor incidence in offspring of pregnant and lactating mice.

Reddy, B. S., "Chemoprevention of Colon Cancer by Dietary Fatty Acids," *Cancer and Metastasis Reviews,* 13, Nos. 3–4 (1994):285–302.

Metabolic, human epidemiological, and laboratory animal studies show enhancement of colon cancer by dietary fat and protection by certain dietary fibers.

Reynolds, R. D., "Vitamin Supplements: Current Controversies," *Journal of the American College of Nutrition,* 13, No. 2 (1994):118–26.

In an area of great controversy, this article presents evidence from recent studies that led the author to conclude that supplementation may be effective in the prevention of cancer, heart disease, neural-tube defects, and other illnesses.

Rohan, T. E., Howe, G. R., Friedenreich, C. M., Jain, M., and Miller, A. B., "Dietary Fiber, Vitamins A, C, and E, and Risk of Breast Cancer: A Cohort Study," *Cancer Causes and Control,* 4, No. 1 (1993):29–37.

Women in the uppermost quintile of dietary fiber intake had a 30 percent lower risk of breast cancer compared with women in the lowest quintile. Similar findings were obtained for intake of pasta, cereals, and vegetables rich in vitamins A and C.

Sandstrom, B., Astrup, A. V., Dyerberg, J., Holmer, G., Poulsen, H. E., Stender, S., Kondrup, J., Gudmand-Hoyer, E., Hlmer, G., and Gudmand-Hyer, E., ["The Effect on Health of Dietary Antioxidants and Antioxidant Supplements"],

Ugeskrift Laeger, 156, No. 51 (1994):7675–79. (Published in Danish, English summary from Medline.)

The authors present evidence that a diet high in fruits and vegetables contains the elements that protect against cancer, heart disease, and cataracts, and that there is no evidence that supplementation with specific antioxidants (for example, beta-carotene and vitamins C and E) can provide the same protection.

Shike, M., "Diet and Lifestyle in the Prevention of Colorectal Cancer: An Overview," *American Journal of Medicine,* 106, No. 1A (1999):11S–15S; discussion 50S–51S.

This review of the research shows that diet can influence all stages in the progression of colorectal cancer, from initiation to promotion. Although surveys show that we as a nation are preoccupied with nutrition, the average person in the United States is still eating too much fat, too many calories, and too few fruits, vegetables, and whole grains. An increase in the intake of plant foods could have a significant impact on reducing mortality from colorectal cancer.

Stavric, B., "Role of Chemopreventers in Human Diet," *Clinical Biochemistry,* 27, No. 5 (1994):319–32.

A review of recent studies examining the role of various foods and phytochemicals in the prevention of chronic diseases, including cancer.

Steele, V. E., Pereira, M. A., Sigman, C. C., and Kelloff, G. A., "Cancer Chemoprevention Agent Development Strategies for Genistein," *Journal of Nutrition,* 125, No. 3 (1995):713S–16S.

Genistein (from soybeans) significantly reduced experimentally induced precancerous sites in the colons of rats.

Steinmetz, K. A., Kushi, L. H., Bostick, R. M., Folsom, A. R., and Potter, J. D., "Vegetables, Fruit, and Colon Cancer in the Iowa Women's Health Study," *American Journal of Epidemiology,* 139, No. 1 (1994):1–15.

The results of this prospective cohort study of a group of over 40,000 women monitored for 5 years support results of epidemiological studies showing that consumption of vegetables, fruits, fiber, and garlic is associated with a significantly reduced risk (20 to 30 percent) of colon cancer.

Stephens, F. O., "Breast Cancer: Aetiological Factors and Associations (a Possible Protective Role of Phytoestrogens)," *Australian and New Zealand Journal of Surgery,* 67, No. 11 (1997):755–60.

This review of the research suggests that it may be not the consumption of red meat and high-fat dairy products but the absence of certain phytochemicals found only in plants that leads to a relationship between diet and breast cancer. Fiber, lignans, and isoflavonoids may play a preventive role in breast cancer by reducing the potential carcinogenic action of prolonged estrogen activity.

Stephens, F. O., "The Increased Incidence of Cancer of the Pancreas: Is There a Missing Dietary Factor? Can It Be Reversed?" *Australian and New Zealand Journal of Surgery,* 69, No. 5 (1999):331–35.

Pancreatic cancer, along with breast and prostate cancer, is on the increase in Western communities. Tobacco use is a key factor in the increase in this cancer, but the Western diet also seems to be related in the same way that it is to the other cancers. In cultures where the consumption of foods containing phyto-estrogens is high, the incidence of pancreatic cancer, as well as breast and prostate cancer, remains low.

Takahashi, O., "Haemorrhagic Toxicity of a Large Dose of Alpha-, Beta-, Gamma-, and Delta-Tocopherols, Ubiquinone, Beta-Carotene, Retinol Acetate and L-Ascorbic Acid in the Rat," *Food and Chemical Toxicology,* 33, No. 2 (1995):121–28.

Overdoses of beneficial food substances, including antioxidants (which can become pro-oxidants and encourage oxidation and cellular damage at high levels), can be dangerous. The substances listed in the title (some of which can be found in high doses in human dietary supplements) significantly increased the likelihood of hemorrhage in rats.

Tanaka, T., Kojima, T., Kawamori, T., and Mori, H., "Chemoprevention of Digestive Organs Carcinogenesis by Natural Product Protocatechuic Acid," *Cancer,* 75, No. 6S (1995):1433–39.

In animal bioassays, this antioxidative phenolic acid present in fruits, vegetables, and nuts was efficacious in reducing carcinogenic action of experimental carcinogens in the oral cavity, stomach, colon, and liver by inhibition of cell proliferation.

Terry, P., Nyrén, O., and Yuen, J., "Protective Effect of Fruits and Vegetables on Stomach Cancer in a Cohort of Swedish Twins," *International Journal of Cancer,* 76, No. 1 (1998):35–37.

In a group of over 11,000 individuals in the Swedish Twin Registry, consumption of fruits and vegetables was inversely related to the incidence of stomach cancer when the diet/cancer relationship was studied over a period of 25 years.

Thompson, L. U., "Antioxidants and Hormone-Mediated Health Benefits of Whole Grains," *Critical Reviews in Food Science and Nutrition,* 34, Nos. 5–6 (1994):473–97.

This paper discusses the role of phytochemicals found in whole grains in the prevention of heart disease and cancer. The author stresses the need to emphasize the whole grain instead of the refined grain in the diet, since the phytochemicals are more concentrated in the fiber in the outer layers of the grain.

Trock, B., Lanza, E., and Greenwald, P., "Dietary Fiber, Vegetables, and Colon

Cancer: Critical Review and Meta-Analyses of the Epidemiologic Evidence," *Journal of the National Cancer Institute,* 82, No. 8 (1990):650–61.

One of the early analyses of over 50 studies, including both epidemiological and case-control studies, showing that a high-vegetable/high-fiber diet cuts the risk of colon cancer by about 50 percent.

Tsushima, M., Maoka, T., Katsuyama, M., Kozuka, M., Matsuno, T., Tokuda, H., Nishino, H., and Iwashima, A., "Inhibitory Effect of Natural Carotenoids on Epstein-Barr Virus Activation Activity of a Tumor Promoter in Raji Cells: A Screening Study for Anti-Tumor Promoters," *Biological and Pharmaceutical Bulletin,* 18, No. 2 (1995):227–33.

This study found other carotenoids to be even more effective than beta-carotene against the tumor promoter that is activated by the Epstein-Barr virus. The other carotenoids included beta-cryptoxanthin, lutein, and lactucaxanthin, as well as some other xanthins that were toxic at high doses, but not at lower ones that also inhibited activation.

Tzonou, A., Signorello, L. B, Lagiou, P., Wuu, J., Trichopoulos, D., and Trichopoupou, A., "Diet and Cancer of the Prostate: A Case-control Study in Greece," *International Journal of Cancer,* 80, No. 5 (1999):704–8.

Several nutrition-related processes appear to contribute to the development of prostate cancer. When men with confirmed prostate cancer were compared with men with benign prostate hypertrophy, polyunsaturated fats appeared to promote this cancer, while consumption of tomatoes, especially cooked tomatoes, and high vitamin E intake appeared to reduce the risk.

Verhagen, H., Poulsen, H. E., Loft, S., van Poppel, G., Willems, M. I., and van Bladeren, P. J., "Reduction of Oxidative DNA-Damage in Humans by Brussels Sprouts," *Carcinogenesis,* 16, No. 4 (1995):969–70.

Signs of oxidative DNA damage were reduced by 28 percent in humans eating 300 grams (approximately 10 ounces) of brussels sprouts daily over a 3-week period. The authors concluded that their findings supported epidemiological studies that show reduced cancer risk with consumption of cruciferous vegetables.

Wattenberg, L. W., "Inhibition of Carcinogenesis by Minor Dietary Constituents," *Cancer Research,* 52, No. 7 (1992):2085S–91S.

A review and analysis of how phytochemicals may exert their chemopreventive effects.

Wattenberg, L. W., "Chemoprevention of Carcinogenesis by Minor Non-Nutrient Constituents of the Diet" (meeting abstract), *Current Strategies of Cancer Chemoprevention, 13th International Symposium on Cancer,* Sapporo, Japan, July 6–9, 1993, p. 10.

Many non-nutritive compounds in the diet—including terpenes, aromatic isothiocyanates, organosulfur compounds, protease inhibitors, monophenols, flavonoids, tannins, other polyphenols, and inositols—may play an important role in the chemoprevention of cancer.

Wattenberg, L. W., and Coccia, J. B., "Inhibition of 4-(Methylnitrosamino)-1-(3-Pyridyl)-1-Butanone Carcinogenesis in Mice by D-Limonene and Citrus Fruit Oils," *Carcinogenesis*, 12, No. 1 (1991):115–17.

D-Limonene and citrus fruit oils (orange and lemon) inhibited pulmonary adenoma formation and the occurrence of forestomach tumors in mice.

Wei, H., Bowen, R., Cai, Q., Barnes, S., and Wang, Y., "Antioxidant and Antipromotional Effects of the Soybean Isoflavone Genistein," *Proceedings of the Society for Experimental Biology and Medicine*, 208, No. 1 (1995):124–30.

Of the compounds tested, genistein was the most potent inhibitor (50 percent reduction) of experimentally produced mouse skin cancer.

Willet, W. C., "Micronutrients and Cancer Risk," *American Journal of Clinical Nutrition*, 59, No. 5 (1994):1162S–65S.

After reviewing the evidence for cancer-preventive activity in various nutrients, the author concludes, "Although we cannot be certain which compounds are responsible, the evidence is overwhelming that an abundant intake of fruits and vegetables can play an important role in reducing cancer incidence."

Willett, W. C., "Nutrition and Cancer," *Salud Publica De Mexico*, 39, No. 4 (1997): 298–309.

After examining various aspects of the diet-and-cancer relationship, the author concludes that we do not yet understand the details. But there is strong evidence that the risk of many cancers can be substantially reduced by staying physically active and lean, increasing the consumption of plant foods, and avoiding high intakes of red meat, animal fat, and alcohol.

Wynder, E. L., Cohen, L. A., Muscat, J. E., Winters, B., Dwyer, J. T., and Blackburn, G., "Breast Cancer: Weighing the Evidence for a Promoting Role of Dietary Fat," *Journal of the National Cancer Institute*, 89, No. 11 (1997):766–75.

Studies of diet and breast cancer within a similar population of women (e.g., only women in the United States) may fail to detect a relationship for two reasons. First, the methods (surveys, self-reports) used to measure food consumption are open to considerable error and second, the diet is relatively homogeneous within the same population. In the United States the diet is relatively high in fat and there is very little difference in fat consumption between those who have and those who do not have the disease. The weight of the evidence from cross-cultural studies, case-control studies, and animal studies consistently shows that the type and total amount of dietary fat affects the development of postmenopausal cancer at several stages in the carcino-genic process.

Yoshioka, K., Deng, T., Cavigelli, M., and Karin, M., "Antitumor Promotion by Phenolic Antioxidants: Inhibition of AP-1 Activity through Induction of Fra Expression," *Proceedings of the National Academy of Sciences of the United States of America,* 92, No. 11 (1995):4972–76.

This study examined the mechanism by which phenolic antioxidants help ac-tivate enzymes that inhibit the promotion as well as the initiation of tumors.

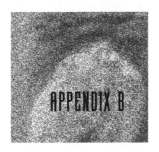

APPENDIX B

Relaxation Training and Meditation

Deep Muscular Relaxation

Deep muscular relaxation is a quick and effective way to achieve both physical and mental relaxation. It works because, with mentally focused training, tensed muscles can become more relaxed than they were prior to the tension. When deep muscular relaxation training is combined with the specific "Breath of Relaxation" that I will also show you how to do, you can achieve almost instantaneous physical and mental relief.

Training begins by tensing and relaxing various sets of muscles throughout your body. This will enable you to experience the relaxed state you are aiming for. You will no longer need to tense your muscles before relaxing them after only two or three days of practice. You will simply use the Breath of Relaxation to instantaneously lessen tension in any region of the body that needs it. At the same time you clear your mind for a few moments, and then make a new beginning at whatever you were doing.

You will need to set aside about 20 minutes over each of the next few days for practice. You should be sitting in a comfortable chair, with or without arms, in a quiet place where you will not be disturbed. If your chair has no arms, rest your hands in your lap, except when the exercise calls for hand movements.

When you tense your muscles during training, go only to about three-quarters of their maximum tension. More is not needed. Do each exercise twice, relax for 5 or 10 seconds in between, then proceed to the next.

You can do these exercises with your eyes open or closed, but you will probably be more focused and relaxed afterward if you do them with your eyes closed. Remember to breathe normally throughout, except in the special breathing exercise.

THE DEEP MUSCULAR RELAXATION TRAINING ROUTINE

1. Make a fist with your right hand. Hold it for 5 seconds, focusing on the tension in the muscles in your hand and up your arm. Relax, and note the difference between the tension and the relaxation.
2. Make fists with both hands. Hold for 5 seconds, noting feelings in the muscles involved. Relax.

    Always remember to focus on the difference in the feelings in your muscles; contrast the feeling of the tension with the feeling as you let go and relax. It helps to think "Let go" as you relax.
3. Make fists with both hands and slowly raise your forearms up to your shoulders, imagining that you are lifting fairly heavy weights. Hold for 5 seconds, then relax ("let go") and return your arms to the resting position.

    The next 7 exercises are for the head, neck, and shoulders, which are focal points for tension in most people.

4. Raise your eyebrows as far as you can. Hold for 5 seconds. Relax.
5. Crease your forehead (bringing your eyebrows together). Hold for 5 seconds. Relax.
6. Press your lips together. Hold for 5 seconds. Relax.
7. Scrunch up your whole face (make a funny face; it doesn't matter exactly how, just as long as you feel some tension in several muscle areas of your face). Hold for 5 seconds. Relax.
8. Lean your head to the right (without adding any special tension). Just note the naturally occurring tension on the sides of your neck as you do this. Hold for 5 seconds. Relax. Repeat the exercise leaning to the left. Then repeat leaning forward, bringing your chin toward your chest.

    (Remember to keep breathing normally. And take your time—don't rush through these exercises!)
9. Raise your shoulders toward your ears (without adding any special tension). Hold for 5 seconds. Relax.
10. Shrug your shoulders—that is, bring them as far forward and toward each other in front of your chest as you can. Hold for 5 seconds. Relax.

The next exercise is the **Breath of Relaxation.**

11. Take a deep breath by first expanding your stomach area, then mid-chest, and finally upper chest so that your lungs are filled to their maximum. Note the tension that occurs naturally in your upper body. Hold your breath for a count of 5 and exhale, letting loose in your neck, shoulders, upper arms, and anywhere else that you noted any tension. Repeat this exercise with particular attention to "letting go" as you exhale.

    You can practice this exercise by itself, several times a day. With just a small amount of practice you will be able to "let go" and relax any time you need to. Just take a deep breath, and consciously release tension in your upper body as you exhale. Besides being an almost instantaneous release of tension, it clears your mind for a few moments of mental relaxation.

The next 3 exercises are for your midsection.

12. Tense your stomach muscles as though to protect yourself from a blow to your midsection. Hold for 5 seconds. Relax.
13. Press your back against your chair. Hold for 5 seconds. Relax.
14. Squeeze your buttocks together. Hold for 5 seconds. Relax.

The next set of 3 exercises is for your lower body.

15. Press your knees together. Hold for 5 seconds. Relax.
16. Press your heels down against the floor. Hold for 5 seconds. Relax.
17. Pull your toes back toward the soles of your feet. Hold for 5 seconds. Relax.

Finish the entire relaxation training exercise by repeating the Breath of Relaxation twice. Then let your attention focus on the feeling in various parts of your body. Start with your head and work down. If you feel any residual tension in any part of your body, give that part a little wiggle and consciously "let go."

Sit quietly for a few moments, breathe normally, and then open your eyes if they have been closed. You are ready to resume your regular daily activities.

With a couple of days' practice the sense of how your body feels when it is relaxed will be in your mind and under mental control. You will no longer need to tense your muscles before directing them to relax. Just take a deep breath, exhale, and let go in whatever part of your body you felt any tension. If you are like most people, you probably experience a certain amount of tension in your head, neck, and shoulder regions, which, fortunately, are the regions most easily controlled and relaxed with the Breath of Relaxation exercise.

Meditation

Although there are a number of different forms of meditation, all focus on breathing and some relaxing mental procedure. Whichever specific way you choose can, with practice, have beneficial physical and mental effects, including the lowering of blood pressure, heart rate, and respiration rate, as well as clearing of the mind.

Here is a simple but effective meditation technique that you can learn quite easily. I think you will experience a great deal of satisfaction the very first time you practice it.

Go to a quiet place where you can sit comfortably without being disturbed. Use an armchair if possible, so you can support your elbows and let your hands rest comfortably in your lap.

Close your eyes.

Check out your body.

If you feel any tension in your neck and shoulders, just rotate your head easily and slowly first in one direction, then the other, a couple of times. Wiggle your shoulders.

Focus on your breathing. Breathe slowly and naturally.

Quiet your mind by focusing in one of the following ways:

Pay attention only to the physical experience of breathing as you slowly inhale—that is, your chest expanding, the feeling of the air flowing in through your nostrils.

Make some sort of sound, mentally, or repeat a word, mentally, as you slowly exhale—for example, "uhmmmm," the word "one," or any other word, phrase, or prayer that, because of its meaning in your life, has a calming effect.

Should outside thoughts intrude, as they probably will, especially when you first begin to practice meditation, just pull back and distance yourself from them. Simply notice them as though they came from someplace outside yourself. It's very important to stay quiet and relaxed, and never to feel that anything you experience while meditating is somehow "wrong" or that you are not doing it "right." Even if you find yourself doing it many times, this act of putting yourself at a distance from any intrusion—becoming completely dispassionate no matter what your mind happens to do, and returning to your word or phrase and calm rhythmic breathing—is a key to experiencing the benefits of meditation.

If you spend about 20 minutes in meditation each day I think you will find that a feeling of calmness and of being in control will spread to other aspects of your life.

Here are some variations that you might enjoy in your meditation:

1. Count slowly to 4 as you breathe in and to a count of either 4 or 6 as you breathe out. Some people find it more relaxing to breathe out more slowly than in, but it's up to you to decide what feels best to you.
2. Instead of a word or counting as you breathe, just establish a calm rhythm, and simply listen. Don't do anything but listen to all the sounds around you. Focus on your breathing and your ears. When thoughts intrude, as they will, do the distancing exercise and return to listening. This meditation approach involves different parts of the brain than when you repeat sounds to yourself (a word or phrase). I find it particularly relaxing.
3. "Meditation in motion is superior to meditation at rest," according to one Oriental teacher of meditation. If you can walk or jog in a safe place where you don't have to pay attention to traffic, dogs, or other distractions, get into a steady rhythm and count your steps as you breathe in and out (for example, breathe in for 4 steps and out for 4 steps). Or simply switch into your "listening" mode and listen to what's going on around you. It's important with meditation in motion only that you have a rhythm in your motion. I have known runners and swimmers who go into an almost trance-like state during activity, but you have to be able to do the activity easily and without paying it any attention.

With meditation in motion you obtain the benefits of two activities—you burn many extra calories and end up being greatly relaxed. It's a great way to combat stress.

I strongly encourage you to experiment with one of the stress-management approaches that I have described in this appendix. Almost everyone who does finds at least one aspect of the techniques to be helpful. Within a matter of a couple of days that particular aspect of your practice, either the Breath of Relaxation or a mental "letting go" such as you experience while meditating, will automatically replace the physical and mental reactions that, up to now, have been your response to stressful events. You will appear to others, as well as to yourself, as a different person. You will be conveying to others that you are in control, and their interactions with you will change. That may be all it takes to alter interpersonal situations that have been responsible for some of the stress in your life.

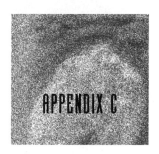

Recipe Analyses:
Fat, Calories, and Fiber

The analyses for total fat, calories, and fiber in the alphabetical listing below are per serving (the larger serving size if a range is given), using the first-named ingredient when alternatives are suggested and without optional ingredients. Except for cheese, optional ingredients add little fat or calories to the analysis. If you add optional cheese, look up the amount used in the Fat and Fiber Counter (Appendix D) and add it to the analysis below.

RECIPE	TOTAL FAT, CALORIES, AND FIBER
Artichoke and Crabmeat Salad	5 g. fat, 147 calories, 7 g. fiber
Asparagus and Pine Nuts	6 g. fat, 73 calories, 2 g. fiber
Baked Fish Fillets	5 g. fat, 168 calories, 0 g. fiber
Baked Swordfish	8 g. fat, 187 calories, 0 g. fiber
Banana Muffins	4 g. fat, 182 calories, 3 g. fiber
Barley and Vegetables	5 g. fat, 138 calories, 5 g. fiber
Barley/Pine-Nut Casserole	6 g. fat, 190 calories, 5 g. fiber
Basic Pancake Mix	3 g. fat, 67 calories, 0 g. fiber
Basic Vinaigrette	9 g. fat, 84 calories, 0 g. fiber
Beet and Cabbage Borscht	2 g. fat, 48 calories, 1 g. fiber
Black Beans and Chili Tomatoes	1 g. fat, 169 calories, 11 g. fiber
Black-Eyed Peas and Greens	3 g. fat, 194 calories, 6 g. fiber
Bok Choy and Mushrooms	4 g. fat, 48 calories, 1 g. fiber
Brancakes	1 g. fat, 195 calories, 5 g. fiber

RECIPE	TOTAL FAT, CALORIES, AND FIBER
Broccoflower Puree	1 g. fat, 45 calories, 2 g. fiber
Broccoli Salad	8 g. fat, 121 calories, 2 g. fiber
Broccoli Walnut Stir-Fry	18 g. fat, 248 calories, 5 g. fiber
Broiled Chicken with Yogurt	13 g. fat, 275 calories, 0 g. fiber
Brownies	3 g. fat, 105 calories, 2 g. fiber
Brown Rice with Garlic	3 g. fat, 211 calories, 2 g. fiber
Brussels Sprouts with Garlic and Oil	3 g. fat, 75 calories, 6 g. fiber
Burneta's Millet Mash	3 g. fat, 248 calories, 4 g. fiber
Cabbage, Carrot, Green Pepper, and Raisin Salad	7 g. fat, 102 calories, 2 g. fiber
Caramel Brownies	2 g. fat, 82 calories, 1 g. fiber
Carrots and Celery	1 g. fat, 41 calories, 2 g. fiber
Cauliflower du Barry	2 g. fat, 83 calories, 3 g. fiber
Celery Soup	3 g. fat, 59 calories, 1 g. fiber
Chewy Cocoa Cake with Quick Chocolate Frosting	4 g. fat, 188 calories, 3 g. fiber
Chicken, Chard, and Rice Soup	9 g. fat, 228 calories, 3 g. fiber
Chicken, Rice, and Artichoke Salad	7 g. fat, 106 calories, 2 g. fiber
Chilled Tomato-Orange Soup with Avocado	8 g. fat, 127 calories, 3 g. fiber
Clam Chowder	1 g. fat, 113 calories, 1 g. fiber
Cold Cucumber Soup	6 g. fat, 119 calories, 2 g. fiber
Confetti Pasta with Fish and Artichokes	9 g. fat, 303 calories, 5 g. fiber
Corncakes	6 g. fat, 289 calories, 4 g. fiber
Couscous, Chickpeas, and Vegetables	3 g. fat, 166 calories, 4 g. fiber
Creamy Cabbage	3 g. fat, 69 calories, 2 g. fiber
Creamy Tofu Dressing	2 g. fat, 27 calories, 0 g. fiber
Creole Stew	2 g. fat, 63 calories, fiber NA
Cucumber/Cabbage/Tomato Salad	4 g. fat, 97 calories, 2 g. fiber
Curried Chicken and Spinach (with Rice)	14 g. fat, 463 calories, 6 g. fiber
Curried Chickpeas and Potatoes	7 g. fat, 359 calories, 9 g. fiber
Curried Squash/Cauliflower Soup	6 g. fat, 124 calories, 4 g. fiber
Curried Tofu and Cabbage	5 g. fat, 108 calories, 5 g. fiber
Dark Chocolate Cheesecake	7 g. fat, 168 calories, 1 g. fiber
Dave's Hearty Meat Sauce	9 g. fat, 202 calories, 3 g. fiber
Dave's Rich and Zesty Burritos	6 g. fat, 192 calories, 5 g. fiber
Dave's Rich and Zesty Tostados	4 g. fat, 175 calories, 6 g. fiber
Dusty Cauliflower	8 g. fat, 118 calories, 3 g. fiber
Eggplant Salad	5 g. fat, 91 calories, 4 g. fiber

Enid's Quick Fruit Pie	4 g. fat, 154 calories, 1 g. fiber
Escarole Torte	7 g. fat, 113 calories, 2 g. fiber
French Toast	4 g. fat, 210 calories, 4 g. fiber
Fresh Beets	4 g. fat, 122 calories, 6 g. fiber
Garlic Vinaigrette	10 g. fat, 93 calories, 0 g. fiber
Gazpacho Primo	3 g. fat, 76 calories, 2 g. fiber
Greek Couscous Salad	7 g. fat, 135 calories, 2 g. fiber
Green-Bean Casserole	4 g. fat, 128 calories, 6 g. fiber
Green-Bean Ragout	8 g. fat, 205 calories, 6 g. fiber
Herbed Potatoes	5 g. fat, 138 calories, 2 g. fiber
Honey-Apricot Bread	1 g. fat, 120 calories, 2 g. fiber
Lee's Power Breakfast	17 g. fat, 488 calories, 15 g. fiber
Lemon and Garlic Dressing	10 g. fat, 92 calories, 0 g. fiber
Main-Course Greek Salad	7 g. fat, 89 calories, 1 g. fiber
Meatless Meat Loaf	3 g. fat, 194 calories, fiber NA
Mediterranean-Style Spinach	5 g. fat, 87 calories, 4 g. fiber
Mexican Quinoa Salad	5 g. fat, 134 calories, 4 g. fiber
Mock Lasagna	8 g. fat, 281 calories, 4 g. fiber
Monna's White Chili	9 g. fat, 298 calories, 1 g. fiber
Mushroom Soup	3 g. fat, 103 calories, 1 g. fiber
Nutty Pepper Pasta	17 g. fat, 368 calories, 5 g. fiber
Once-a-Week Pasta	9 g. fat, 354 calories, 6 g. fiber
Onion Gravy	1 g. fat, 21 calories, 0 g. fiber
Onion Quiche	7 g. fat, 163 calories, 2 g. fiber
Orange Roughy with Spinach	5 g. fat, 184 calories, 2 g. fiber
Oven-Fried Chicken	12 g. fat, 356 calories, 1 g. fiber
Oven-Stewed Chicken and Vegetables	4 g. fat, 350 calories, 8 g. fiber
Parmesan-Dill Brussels Sprouts	3 g. fat, 77 calories, 6 g. fiber
Pasta Salad	5 g. fat, 170 calories, 4 g. fiber
Pasta with Garlic-Clam Sauce	10 g. fat, 382 calories, 3 g. fiber
Pickled Beets	0 g. fat, 49 calories, 2 g. fiber
Potato-Tofu Casserole	12 g. fat, 237 calories, 4 g. fiber
Rainbow Salad	5 g. fat, 138 calories, 2 g. fiber
Roasted Onion Salad	9 g. fat, 124 calories, 2 g. fiber
Roasted Rosemary Potatoes	4 g. fat, 139 calories, 2 g. fiber
Roasted Vegetables	5 g. fat, 111 calories, 4 g. fiber
Roast Pork Tenderloin	5 g. fat, 169 calories, 0 g. fiber
Roast Poultry, Tandoori Style (with white meat)	1 g. fat, 119 calories, 0 g. fiber

Recipe	Total Fat, Calories, and Fiber
Roast Poultry, Tandoori Style (with dark meat)	6 g. fat, 159 calories, 0 g. fiber
Rosemary Carrots	1 g. fat, 47 calories, 2 g. fiber
Savory Turkey Loaf	5 g. fat, 255 calories, 4 g. fiber
Scalloped Potatoes and Tofu	7 g. fat, 153 calories, 2 g. fiber
Seafood Stove-Top Casserole	2 g. fat, 132 calories, 1 g. fiber
Shredded Cabbage and Carrot Salad	4 g. fat, 59 calories, 1 g. fiber
Simple Pot of Beans	1 g. fat, 116 calories, 6 g. fiber
Soup of the Day	2 g. fat, 196 calories, 8 g. fiber
Southwest Casserole	12 g. fat, 337 calories, 2 g. fiber
Soybean and Lima Casserole	4 g. fat, 181 calories, 8 g. fiber
Spaghetti with Tomatoes, Basil, and Capers	15 g. fat, 424 calories, 5 g. fiber
Spiced Tofu Loaf	8 g. fat, 134 calories, 2 g. fiber
Spinach Casserole	7 g. fat, 209 calories, 6 g. fiber
Spinach Lasagna	16 g. fat, 405 calories, 4 g. fiber
Steak Marinade, Basic	5 g. fat, 157 calories, 2 g. fiber
Steak Marinade, Oriental	5 g. fat, 174 calories, 2 g. fiber
Stuffed Winter Squash	5 g. fat, 334 calories, 10 g. fiber
Tamale Pie	7 g. fat, 232 calories, 7 g. fiber
Tarragon Chicken Salad with Vermicelli	5 g. fat, 198 calories, 7 g. fiber
Teriyaki Salmon	13 g. fat, 271 calories, 0 g. fiber
Three-Bean Salad	14 g. fat, 192 calories, 5 g. fiber
Tri-Color Pepper Sauté	6 g. fat, 86 calories, 1 g. fiber
Tuna Casserole	5 g. fat, 227 calories, 2 g. fiber
Tuna with Chickpeas	9 g. fat, 293 calories, 5 g. fiber
Whole-Wheat Coffee Cake	4 g. fat, 123 calories, 1 g. fiber
Zucchini Boats	2 g. fat, 26 calories, 1 g. fiber

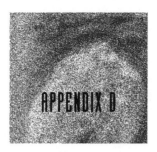

Fat and Fiber Counter and Daily Eating Diary

How to Use the Counter

The food items listed in this counter are in alphabetical order within several different food categories.[1]

Included are a number of new lower-fat foods and combination foods, some listed by manufacturer and some as averages from several manufacturers without naming them. Values for homemade (hmde) combination foods such as soups, salads, and sandwiches represent combinations of ingredients from traditional recipes.

I do not list fast-food chains since complete nutritional listings are either posted or available for the asking at these establishments. In general, the lowest-fat items at fast-food restaurants are grilled chicken sandwiches, plain hamburgers, or roast beef sandwiches (all without cheese or dressing), salads with low-fat dressings, and frozen yogurt for dessert. Avoid fried foods.

I list fat values for extra lean, lean, regular, high fat, and highest fat among the meats, but you should understand that the "extra-lean" and "lean" cuts are for expertly trimmed portions prepared expressly for laboratory analysis. They are as devoid of fat as you can get. Many super-

---

[1]Data for the counter are drawn from *The T-Factor Fat Gram Counter* by Jamie Pope, M.S., R.D., and Martin Katahn, Ph.D. (New York: W. W. Norton, 1996), which contains additional information and entries.

markets and independent butchers may leave a certain amount of fat on the meats they call "extra lean" or "lean," so it's up to you to do some trimming at home if you want your meats to approximate the values given for "extra lean" and "lean" in this counter.

Food values are listed in commonly used portions. Information is given for total fat, calories, and fiber.

Instructions for keeping a daily eating diary, with a sample page, appear at the end of the counter.

Organization of the Counter

The categories of food are organized as follows, with the page numbers of their beginnings.

Item	Serving	Total Fat (g)	Calories	Fiber (g)
Beverages				
apple juice	6 fl. oz.	0	90	0
beer				
regular*	12 fl. oz.	0	148	0
light*	12 fl. oz.	0	100	0
nonalcoholic	12 fl. oz.	0	90	0
carbonated drink				
regular	12 fl. oz.	0	152	0
sugar free	12 fl. oz.	0	1	0
club soda/seltzer	12 fl. oz.	0	0	0
coffee, brewed				
or instant	8 fl. oz.	0	4	0
coffee, flavored mixes,				
instant	6 fl. oz.	2.4	55	0
cordials and liqueurs,				
54 proof*	1 fl. oz.	0	97	0
daiquiri*	3.5 fl. oz.	0	122	0
eggnog,				
nonalcoholic				
w/whole milk	8 fl. oz.	19.0	342	0
w/2% milk	8 fl. oz.	8.1	188	0
gin, 90 proof*	1 fl. oz.	0	70	0
lemonade, mix or				
frzn	8 fl. oz.	0	102	0
lemonade,				
sugar-free	8 fl. oz.	0	4	0
orange juice,				
unsweetened	6 fl. oz.	0	83	0
pineapple-orange juice	6 fl. oz.	0	99	0
rum, 80 proof*	1 fl. oz.	0	70	0
tea, brewed or instant	8 fl. oz.	0	0	0
tonic water	8 fl. oz.	0	90	0
vodka, 80 proof*	1 fl. oz.	0	70	0
whiskey, 86 proof*	1 fl. oz.	0	70	0
wine*				
dessert and apertif	4 fl. oz.	0	184	0
red or rosé	4 fl. oz.	0	85	0
white, dry or				
medium	4 fl. oz.	0	80	0
wine cooler	8 fl. oz.	0	83	0
Breads and Flours				
bagel, cinnamon raisin	1 medium	2.0	240	2
bagel, plain	1 medium	1.4	180	2
barley flour	1 cup	3.0	600	31
biscuit				
baking powder	1 medium	6.6	156	1
buttermilk	1 medium	4.8	103	1
from mix	1 medium	4.3	121	1
bread				
cracked wheat	1 slice	1.0	65	1
French/Vienna	1 slice	1.0	70	1
honey wheatberry	1 slice	1.1	70	2
Italian	1 slice	0.5	78	1

Item	Serving	Total Fat (g)	Calories	Fiber (g)
mixed grain	1 slice	0.9	70	2
multigrain, "lite"	1 slice	0.5	45	3
pita, plain	1 large	0.8	240	2
pita, whole wheat	1 large	1.2	236	7
raisin	1 slice	1.0	70	1
Roman meal	1 slice	1.0	70	1
rye, American	1 slice	0.9	66	2
rye, pumpernickel	1 slice	0.8	82	2
sourdough	1 slice	1.0	70	1
wheat, commercial	1 slice	1.0	70	1
wheat, "lite"	1 slice	0.5	45	3
white, commercial	1 slice	1.0	70	0
white, hmde	1 slice	1.7	72	0
white, "lite"	1 slice	0.5	42	2
whole wheat,				
commercial	1 slice	1.2	80	2
breadcrumbs	1 cup	4.6	392	3
breadsticks				
plain	1 small	0.3	39	0
sesame	1 small	2.2	51	0
bulgur, dry	1 cup	2.0	477	25
cornbread				
from mix	⅛ mix	4.0	160	1
hmde	1 piece	7.3	198	2
cornmeal, dry	1 cup	1.6	502	10
cornstarch	1 T	0	35	0
crackers				
cheese	5 pieces	4.9	81	0
Cheese Nips	13 crackers	3.0	70	0
cheese w/peanut				
butter	2-oz. pkg.	13.5	283	0
Goldfish, any flavor	12 crackers	2.0	34	0
graham	2 squares	1.3	60	0
graham, crumbs	½ cup	4.5	180	2
Harvest Wheats	4 crackers	3.6	72	0
Hi Ho	4 crackers	4.0	70	0
matzohs	1 board	1.9	115	0
melba toast	1 piece	0.1	15	0
Norwegian				
flatbread	2 thin	0.3	40	0
oyster	33 crackers	3.3	109	0
rice cakes	1 piece	0.2	35	0
Ritz	3 crackers	3.0	53	0
rye w/cheese	1.5-oz. pkg.	9.5	205	0
Ryekrisp, plain	2 crackers	0.2	40	0
Ryekrisp, sesame	2 crackers	1.4	60	0
saltines	2 crackers	0.6	26	0
sesame wafers	3 crackers	3.0	70	0
Snackwell's cheese	18 crackers	1.0	60	0
Snackwell's wheat	5 crackers	0.0	50	1
soda	5 crackers	1.9	63	0
Triscuit	2 crackers	1.3	42	0
Vegetable Thins	7 crackers	4.0	70	0
Wasa crispbread	1 piece	1.0	45	1

*Although alcohol contains no fat, scientific evidence suggests that it may facilitate fat storage and hamper efforts to lose weight. Excessive alcohol intake is detrimental to your health. I concur with other health organizations in recommending discretion in the use of alcoholic beverages.

Item	Serving	Total Fat (g)	Calories	Fiber (g)
Wheat Thins	4 crackers	1.5	35	0
Wheatsworth	5 crackers	3.0	70	0
zwieback	2 crackers	1.2	60	0
crepe	1 medium	1.5	48	0
croissant	1 medium	11.5	167	1
croutons, commercial	¼ cup	2.2	59	1
Danish pastry	1 medium	19.3	256	1
doughnut				
cake	1 2.2 oz.	16.2	250	1
yeast	1 2.2 oz.	13.3	235	1
English muffin				
plain	1	1.1	135	1
w/raisins	1	1.2	150	1
whole wheat	1	2.6	170	2
flour				
buckwheat	1 cup	3.0	328	8
carob	1 cup	1.0	394	13
rice	1 cup	1.3	428	3
rye, medium	1 cup	2.2	400	13
soy	1 cup	18.0	380	2
wheat, cake	1 cup	0.9	436	4
white, all purpose	1 cup	1.4	499	4
white, bread	1 cup	3.0	401	4
white, self-rising	1 cup	1.2	436	4
whole wheat	1 cup	2.4	400	11
French toast				
frzn variety	1 slice	6.0	139	0
hmde	1 slice	10.7	172	1
hushpuppy	1 medium	5.5	153	1
matzoh ball	1	7.6	121	0
muffins				
all types, commercial	1 large (3 oz.)	10.3	242	1
bran, hmde	1 medium	5.1	112	2
corn	1 medium	4.2	130	1
white, plain	1 medium	4.0	118	0
pancakes				
blueberry, from mix	3 medium	15.0	320	4
buckwheat, from mix	3 medium	12.3	270	3
buttermilk, from mix	3 medium	10.0	270	2
hmde	3 medium	9.6	312	2
"lite," from mix	3 medium	2.0	190	5
whole-wheat, from mix	3 medium	3.0	180	6
pie crust, plain	⅛ pie	8.0	125	0
rice bran	1 oz.	0.4	80	2
rolls				
brown & serve	1	2.2	100	0
crescent	1	5.6	102	1
croissant	1 small	6.0	120	0
French	1	0.4	137	1
hamburger	1	3.0	180	1
hard	1	1.2	115	1
hot dog	1	2.1	116	1
kaiser/hoagie	1 medium	2.0	190	1
parkerhouse	1	2.1	59	0
rye, dark	1	1.6	55	2
rye, light, hard	1	1.0	79	2

Item	Serving	Total Fat (g)	Calories	Fiber (g)
sesame seed	1	2.1	59	1
sourdough	1	1.0	100	1
submarine	1 medium	3.0	290	2
wheat	1	0.8	72	1
white, commercial	1	2.0	80	0
white, hmde	1	3.1	119	1
whole wheat	1	1.1	85	3
yeast, sweet	1	7.9	198	1
scone	1	5.5	120	1
soft pretzel	1 medium	1.7	190	1
stuffing				
bread, from mix	½ cup	12.2	198	0
cornbread, from mix	½ cup	4.8	175	0
sweet roll, iced	1 medium	7.9	198	1
toaster pastry, any flavor	1	5.0	200	0
tortilla				
corn (unfried)	1 medium	1.1	67	1
flour	1 medium	2.5	85	1
Candy				
butterscotch				
candy	6 pieces	1.0	113	0
chips	1 oz.	6.7	234	0
candied fruit				
apricot	1 oz.	0.1	94	1
cherry	1 oz.	0.1	96	1
citrus peel	1 oz.	0.1	90	1
figs	1 oz.	0.1	84	2
candy-coated almonds	1 oz.	2.0	120	1
caramels				
plain or choc. w/nuts	1 oz.	4.6	120	0
plain or choc. w/o nuts	1 oz.	3.0	110	0
carob-coated raisins	½ cup	13.5	387	5
choc. chips				
milk choc.	¼ cup	11.0	218	1
semi-sweet	¼ cup	12.2	220	1
choc.-covered mint patty	1 small	1.0	40	0
choc.-covered peanuts	1 oz.	11.7	159	2
choc.-covered raisins	1 oz.	14.9	120	1
choc. kisses	6 pieces	9.0	154	1
choc. stars	7 pieces	8.1	160	1
Cracker Jack	1 cup	3.3	170	2
English toffee	1 oz.	2.8	113	0
fudge				
choc.	1 oz.	3.4	112	0
choc. w/nuts	1 oz.	4.9	119	0
gumdrops	28 pieces	0.2	97	0
Gummy Bears	1 oz.	0.1	110	0
hard candy	6 pieces	0.3	108	0
jelly beans	1 oz.	0	104	0
licorice	1 oz.	0.1	35	0
Life Savers	5 pieces	0.1	39	0
malted-milk balls	1 oz.	7.1	137	1
marshmallow	1 large	0	25	0

Item	Serving	Total Fat (g)	Calories	Fiber (g)
marshmallow creme	1 oz.	0.1	88	0
mints	14 pieces	0.6	104	0
peanut brittle	1 oz.	7.7	149	1
Peppermint Pattie	1 oz.	4.8	124	1
Praline	1 oz.	6.9	130	0
Sour balls	1 oz.	0	110	0
taffy	1 oz.	1.5	99	0
yogurt-covered peanuts	½ cup	26.0	387	4
yogurt-covered raisins	½ cup	14.0	313	2

Cereals

Item	Serving	Total Fat (g)	Calories	Fiber (g)
All Bran	⅓ cup	0.5	70	10
Alpha-Bits	1 cup	0.6	111	1
Apple Jacks	1 cup	0.1	110	1
bran, 100%	½ cup	1.9	84	9
bran, unprocessed, dry	¼ cup	0.6	29	6
Bran Buds	⅓ cup	0.7	72	10
Bran Chex	1 cup	1.2	136	9
Bran Flakes, 40%	1 cup	0.7	127	6
Cap'n Crunch	¾ cup	3.4	121	0
Cheerios	1 cup	1.6	90	2
Cocoa Krispies	1 cup	0.5	140	0
Corn Chex	1 cup	0.1	111	1
cornflakes	1 cup	0.1	108	1
corn grits w/o added fat	½ cup	0.5	71	1
Cracklin' Oat Bran	⅓ cup	2.7	72	3
Cream of Wheat w/o added fat	½ cup	0.3	67	0
Crispix	1 cup	0	110	1
Fiber One	1 cup	2.2	128	21
Fiberwise	⅔ cup	1.0	90	5
Frosted Bran, Kelloggs	¾ cup	0	100	3
Fruit & Fibre w/dates, raisins, walnuts	⅔ cup	2.0	120	5
w/peaches, almonds	⅔ cup	2.0	120	5
Fruitful Bran	⅔ cup	0	120	5
Golden Grahams	¾ cup	1.1	109	1
granola commercial brands	⅓ cup	4.9	126	3
hmde	⅓ cup	10.0	184	2
low-fat, Kelloggs	⅓ cup	2.0	120	2
Grapenut Flakes	1 cup	0.4	116	2
Grapenuts	¼ cup	0.1	105	2
Honeynut Cheerios	¾ cup	0.7	107	1
Kix	1½ cup	0.7	110	0
Life, plain or cinn.	1 cup	2.5	152	4
Most	⅔ cup	0.3	95	2
Mueslix, Kellogg's	½ cup	1.0	140	4
Nutri-Grain, Kellogg's almond raisin	⅔ cup	2.0	140	3
raisin bran	1 cup	1.0	130	5
wheat	⅔ cup	0.3	90	3
oat bran, cooked cereal w/o added fat	½ cup	0.5	50	2
oat bran, dry	¼ cup	1.6	82	3

Item	Serving	Total Fat (g)	Calories	Fiber (g)
oats instant	1 packet	1.7	108	1
w/o added fat	½ cup	1.2	72	1
Product 19	1 cup	0.2	108	1
puffed rice	1 cup	0	56	0
puffed wheat	1 cup	0.1	44	1
Raisin Bran	1 cup	0.8	156	5
Rice Chex	1 cup	0.1	110	1
Rice Krispies	1 cup	0.2	110	0
shredded wheat	1 cup	0.3	85	2
Shredded Wheat Squares, fruit filled	½ cup	0	90	3
Special K	1 cup	0.1	111	0
Team	1 cup	0.5	111	1
Total	1 cup	0.7	100	2
Total raisin bran	1 cup	1.0	140	5
Wheat Chex	1 cup	1.2	169	6
wheat germ, toasted	¼ cup	3.0	108	4
Wheaties	1 cup	0.5	99	2
whole-wheat, natural, w/o added fat	½ cup	0.5	75	2

Cheeses

Item	Serving	Total Fat (g)	Calories	Fiber (g)
American processed	1 oz.	8.9	106	0
reduced calorie	1 oz.	2.0	50	0
blue	1 oz.	8.2	100	0
Borden's Fat Free	1 oz.	<0.5	40	0
Borden's Lite Line	1 oz.	2.0	50	0
brick	1 oz.	8.4	105	0
Brie	1 oz.	7.9	95	0
caraway	1 oz.	8.3	107	0
cheddar grated	¼ cup	9.4	114	0
sliced	1 oz.	9.4	114	0
cheese fondue	¼ cup	11.7	170	0
cheese food, cold pack	2 T	7.8	94	0
cheese sauce	¼ cup	9.8	132	0
cheese spread (Kraft)	1 oz.	6.0	82	0
Colby	1 oz.	9.1	112	0
cottage cheese 1% fat	½ cup	1.2	82	0
2% fat	½ cup	2.2	101	0
creamed	½ cup	5.1	117	0
cream cheese Kraft Free	1 oz. (2 T)	0	25	0
"lite" (Neufchâtel)	1 oz. (2 T)	6.6	74	0
regular	1 oz. (2 T)	9.9	99	0
Weight Watchers	1 oz. (2 T)	2.0	35	0
Edam	1 oz.	7.9	101	0
feta	1 oz.	6.0	75	0
Gouda	1 oz.	7.8	101	0
Healthy Choice	1 oz.	0	30	0
hot pepper cheese	1 oz.	6.9	92	0
Jarlsberg	1 oz.	6.9	100	0
Kraft American Singles	1 oz.	7.5	90	0
Kraft Free Singles	1 oz.	0	45	0

Item	Serving	Total Fat (g)	Calories	Fiber (g)
Kraft Light Singles	1 oz.	4.0	70	0
Light n' Lively singles	1 oz.	4.0	70	0
Limburger	1 oz.	7.7	93	0
Monterey Jack	1 oz.	8.6	106	0
mozzarella				
part skim	1 oz.	4.5	72	0
part skim, low				
moisture	1 oz.	4.9	79	0
whole milk	1 oz.	6.1	80	0
whole milk, low				
moisture	1 oz.	7.0	90	0
Muenster	1 oz.	8.5	104	0
Parmesan				
grated	1 T	1.5	23	0
hard	1 oz.	7.3	111	0
Weight Watchers				
Fat Free	1 T	0	14	0
provolone	1 oz.	7.6	100	0
ricotta				
"lite" reduced fat	½ cup	4.0	109	0
part skim	½ cup	9.8	171	0
whole milk	½ cup	16.1	216	0
Romano	1 oz.	7.6	110	0
Roquefort	1 oz.	8.7	105	0
Sargento Preferred Light				
mozzarella	1 oz.	3.0	60	0
Swiss	1 oz.	4.0	80	0
smoked cheese product	1 oz.	7.0	100	0
Swiss				
processed	1 oz.	7.1	95	0
sliced	1 oz.	7.8	107	0

Combination Foods

Item	Serving	Total Fat (g)	Calories	Fiber (g)
baked beans w/pork	½ cup	1.8	134	4
beans				
refried, canned	½ cup	1.4	135	7
refried w/fat	½ cup	13.2	271	7
refried w/sausage,				
canned	½ cup	13.0	194	8
beans & franks,				
canned	1 cup	16.0	366	7
beef & vegetable stew	1 cup	10.5	218	2
beef burgundy	1 cup	21.2	336	1
beef goulash				
w/noodles	1 cup	13.9	335	2
beef stew, canned	1 cup	8.0	184	2
beef teriyaki, Stouffer's	10 oz.	8.0	290	2
beef vegetable stew,				
hmde	1 cup	13.8	244	2
burrito				
bean w/cheese	1 large	11.0	330	4
bean w/o cheese	1 large	3.8	220	4
beef	1 large	19.0	413	2
with guacamole, frzn	6 oz.	16.0	354	2
cannelloni, meat &				
cheese	1 piece	29.7	420	1
casserole, meat, veg.,				
rice, sauce	1 cup	12.2	276	3

Item	Serving	Total Fat (g)	Calories	Fiber (g)
chicken, glazed, Lean				
Cuisine	8½ oz.	8.0	260	1
chicken à la king,				
hmde	1 cup	34.3	468	1
chicken à la king				
w/rice, frzn	1 cup	12.0	360	1
chicken & rice				
casserole	1 cup	18.0	365	1
chicken & veg. stir-fry	1 cup	6.9	142	3
chicken cacciatore,				
Stouffer's	11¼ oz.	11.0	310	1
chicken divan,				
Stouffer's	8½ oz.	20.0	320	0
chicken noodle				
casserole	1 cup	10.7	269	2
chicken parmigiana,				
hmde	7 oz.	14.8	308	2
chicken salad, regular	½ cup	21.2	271	0
chicken tetrazzini	1 cup	19.6	348	1
chili				
w/beans	1 cup	14.8	302	6
w/o beans	1 cup	19.3	302	3
chop suey w/o rice				
beef	1 cup	17.0	300	3
fish or poultry	1 cup	6.7	124	4
chow mein				
beef, canned,				
La Choy	1 cup	2.3	72	2
chicken, canned,				
La Choy	1 cup	2.3	68	2
chicken, hmde	1 cup	8.8	224	2
pepper, La Choy	1 cup	1.4	89	2
crab cake	1 small	3.8	61	0
curry w/o meat	1 cup	6.6	138	2
deviled crab	½ cup	15.4	231	1
deviled egg	1 large	5.3	63	0
egg foo yung w/sauce	1 piece	7.0	129	1
eggplant Parmesan,				
traditional	1 cup	24.0	356	3
egg roll				
frzn, La Choy	4	4.5	112	1
restaurant	1 (3½ oz.)	10.5	153	1
egg salad	½ cup	17.4	212	0
enchilada				
bean, beef, &				
cheese	1 piece	14.1	243	3
beef, frzn	7½ oz.	16.0	250	1
cheese, frzn	8 oz.	21.0	366	1
chicken, frzn	7½ oz.	11.0	247	1
fajitas				
chicken	1	13.5	381	4
beef	1	18.2	302	3
falafel	1 small	5.0	74	1
fettuccine Alfredo	1 cup	29.7	461	1
fillet of fish divan, frzn	12⅜ oz.	3.0	240	0
fish creole	1 cup	5.4	172	2
Hamburger Helper,				
all varieties	1 cup	18.9	375	1

Item	Serving	Total Fat (g)	Calories	Fiber (g)
ham salad w/mayo	½ cup	20.2	277	0
ham spread, Spreadables	½ cup	12.0	180	0
lasagna				
cheese, frzn	10½ oz.	14.0	385	2
hmde w/beef & cheese	1 piece	19.8	400	2
zucchini lasagna, Lean Cuisine	11 oz.	5.0	260	2
lobster				
Cantonese	1 cup	19.6	334	0
Newburg	½ cup	24.8	305	0
salad	½ cup	7.0	119	0
lo mein, Chinese	1 cup	7.2	185	1
macaroni & cheese				
from package	1 cup	17.3	386	0
frzn	6 oz.	12.0	260	0
manicotti, cheese & tomato	1 piece	11.8	238	2
meatball (reg. ground beef)	1 medium	5.1	72	0
meat loaf, w/reg. ground beef	3½ oz.	20.4	332	0
moo goo gai pan	1 cup	17.2	304	1
moussaka	1 cup	8.9	210	3
onion rings	10 average	17.0	234	1
oysters Rockefeller, traditional	6–8 oysters	14.0	230	1
pepper steak	1 cup	11.0	330	1
pizza				
cheese	1 slice	10.1	183	1
cheese, French bread, frzn	5⅛ oz.	13.0	330	1
combination w/meat	1 slice	17.5	272	1
deep dish, cheese	1 slice	13.5	426	4
pepperoni, frzn	¼ pizza	18.0	364	2
pork, sweet & sour, w/rice	1 cup	7.5	270	1
quiche				
Lorraine (bacon)	⅛ pie	43.5	540	1
plain or vegetable	1 slice	17.6	312	1
ratatouille	½ cup	3.0	60	2
salmon patty, traditional	3½ oz.	12.4	239	1
sandwiches				
BBQ beef on bun	1	16.8	392	5
BBQ pork on bun	1	12.2	359	5
BLT w/mayo	1	15.6	282	1
bologna & cheese	1	22.5	363	1
chicken w/mayo & lettuce	1	14.4	303	1
club w/mayo	1	20.8	590	3
corned beef on rye	1	10.8	296	1
cream cheese & jelly	1	16.0	368	1
egg salad	1	12.5	279	1
french dip, au jus	1	12.2	360	2
grilled cheese	1	24.0	426	1
ham, cheese & mayo	1	16.0	350	1
ham salad	1	16.9	321	1
peanut butter & jelly	1	15.1	374	3
Reuben	1	33.3	531	6
roast beef & gravy	1	24.5	429	1
roast beef & mayo	1	22.6	328	1
sub w/salami & cheese	1	41.3	766	3
tuna salad	1	14.2	278	1
turkey & mayo	1	18.4	402	1
turkey breast & mustard	1	5.2	285	1
turkey ham on rye	1	9.0	239	3
shrimp creole w/o rice	1 cup	6.1	146	2
shrimp salad	½ cup	9.5	136	1
spaghetti				
w/meat sauce	1 cup	16.7	317	2
w/red clam sauce	1 cup	7.3	250	2
w/tomato sauce	1 cup	1.5	179	2
w/white clam sauce	1 cup	19.5	416	1
spinach soufflé	1 cup	14.8	212	2
stroganoff				
beef, Stouffer's	9¾ oz.	20.0	390	1
beef w/o noodles	1 cup	44.4	568	1
taco, beef	1 medium	17.0	272	2
tamale w/sauce	1 piece	6.0	114	1
tortellini, meat or cheese	1 cup	15.4	363	1
tostada w/refried beans	1 medium	16.3	294	6
tuna noodle casserole	1 cup	13.3	315	2
tuna salad				
oil pack, w/mayo	½ cup	16.3	226	0
water pack, w/mayo	½ cup	10.5	170	0
veal parmigiana				
frzn	5 oz.	16.2	287	0
hmde	1 cup	25.5	485	2
veal scallopini	1 cup	20.4	429	2
Desserts and Toppings				
apple betty, fruit crisps	½ cup	13.3	347	3
baklava	1 piece	29.2	426	2
brownie				
butterscotch	1	1.8	52	0
choc., "light," from mix	1/24 pkg.	2.0	100	0
choc., plain	1 small	3.4	64	0
cake				
angel food	1/12 cake	0.1	161	0
butter w/frosting	1/12 cake	13.0	380	1
carrot w/frosting	1/12 cake	19.0	420	3
choc. w/frosting	1/12 cake	17.0	388	2
coconut w/frosting	1/12 cake	18.1	395	2
devil's food, "light," from mix	1/12 cake	3.5	190	0
gingerbread	2½" slice	2.9	267	0
lemon w/frosting	1/12 cake	16.0	410	1

Item	Serving	Total Fat (g)	Calories	Fiber (g)
pineapple upside-down	2½" slice	9.1	236	2
pound	1⁄12 cake	9.0	200	1
pound, Entenmann fat-free	1-oz. slice	0	70	0
spice w/frosting	1⁄12 cake	13.5	370	1
sponge	1 piece	3.1	190	0
white w/frosting	1⁄12 cake	14.6	369	1
yellow w/frosting	1⁄12 cake	16.4	391	1
cheesecake, traditional	⅛ pie	22.0	372	0
cobbler				
w/biscuit topping	½ cup	6.0	209	3
w/pie-crust topping	½ cup	9.3	236	3
cookie				
animal	15 cookies	4.7	152	0
anise-seed	1	4.0	63	0
anisette toast	1 slice	1.0	109	0
arrowroot	1	0.9	24	0
choc.	1	3.3	56	0
choc. chip, hmde	1	3.7	68	0
choc. chip, Pepperidge Farm	1	2.5	100	0
choc. sandwich (Oreo type)	1	2.1	49	0
Entenmann's fat-free	2	0	75	0
fat-free Newtons	1	0	70	0
fig bar	1	1.0	56	1
Fig Newtons	1	1.0	60	0
gingersnap	1	1.6	34	0
graham cracker, choc. covered	1	3.1	62	0
macaroon, coconut	1	3.4	60	0
molasses	1	3.0	80	0
oatmeal	1	3.2	80	0
oatmeal, Pepperidge Farm	1 large	6.4	120	1
oatmeal raisin	1	3.0	83	0
peanut butter	1	3.2	72	1
Rice Krispie bar	1	0.9	36	0
shortbread	1	2.3	42	0
Snack Well's				
bite size chocolate chip	6	1.0	60	0
cinnamon graham snacks	9	0	50	0
creme sandwich cookies	1	1.0	50	0
devil's food cookie cakes	1	0	60	0
oatmeal raisin	1	1.0	60	0
Social Tea biscuit	1	0.6	22	0
sugar	1	3.4	89	0
sugar wafers	2 small	2.1	53	0
vanilla-creme sandwich	1	3.1	69	0
vanilla wafers	3	1.8	51	0

Item	Serving	Total Fat (g)	Calories	Fiber (g)
cupcake				
choc. w/icing	1	5.5	159	1
yellow w/icing	1	6.0	160	1
custard, baked	½ cup	6.9	148	0
date bar	1 bar	2.0	90	1
eclair				
w/choc. icing & custard	1 small	15.4	316	0
w/choc. icing & whipped cream	1 small	25.7	296	0
fruitcake	1 piece	6.2	154	1
fruit ice, Italian	½ cup	0	123	0
gelatin				
low-cal.	½ cup	0	8	0
regular, sweetened	½ cup	0	70	0
granola bar	1 bar	6.8	141	1
ice cream				
choc. (10% fat)	½ cup	8.0	150	1
choc. (16% fat)	½ cup	17.0	210	0
dietetic, sugar-free	½ cup	3.5	90	0
French vanilla soft serve	½ cup	11.3	189	0
Simple Pleasures (Simpless)	½ cup	0.5	120	0
strawberry (10% fat)	½ cup	6.0	128	0
vanilla (10% fat)	½ cup	7.2	134	0
vanilla (16% fat)	½ cup	11.9	175	0
Weight Watchers	½ cup	0.8	81	0
ice cream bar				
choc. coated	1 bar	11.5	198	0
toffee krunch	1 bar	10.2	149	1
ice cream cake roll	1 slice	6.9	159	0
ice cream cone (cone only)	1 medium	0.3	45	0
ice cream drumstick	1	10.0	188	1
ice cream sandwich	1	8.3	204	0
ice milk				
choc.	½ cup	2.0	204	0
soft serve, all flavors	½ cup	2.3	112	0
strawberry	½ cup	2.5	100	0
vanilla	½ cup	2.8	92	0
pie				
apple	⅛ pie	16.9	347	3
banana cream or custard	⅛ pie	14.0	353	1
blueberry	⅛ pie	17.3	387	3
Boston cream pie	⅛ pie	10.0	260	1
cherry	⅛ pie	18.1	418	2
choc. meringue, traditional	⅛ pie	18.0	378	1
coconut cream or custard	⅛ pie	19.0	365	1
key lime	⅛ pie	19.0	388	1
lemon chiffon	⅛ pie	13.5	335	1
lemon meringue, traditional	⅛ pie	13.1	350	1
mincemeat	⅛ pie	18.4	434	3
peach	⅛ pie	17.7	421	3

Item	Serving	Total Fat (g)	Calories	Fiber (g)
pecan	⅛ pie	23.0	510	2
pumpkin	⅛ pie	16.8	367	5
raisin	⅛ pie	12.9	325	1
rhubarb	⅛ pie	17.1	405	3
strawberry	⅛ pie	9.1	228	1
sweet potato	⅛ pie	18.2	342	2
pudding				
any flavor except				
choc.	½ cup	4.3	165	0
bread	½ cup	7.4	212	1
choc., D-Zerta	½ cup	0.5	65	0
choc. w/whole milk	½ cup	5.8	220	1
from mix w/skim milk	½ cup	0	124	0
noodle	½ cup	5.3	141	0
rice	½ cup	4.1	175	0
tapioca	½ cup	4.1	161	0
pudding pop, frzn	1 bar	2.0	80	0
sherbet	½ cup	1.0	130	0
soufflé, choc.	½ cup	3.9	63	0
strudel, fruit	½ cup	1.2	47	1
toppings				
butterscotch/caramel	3 T	0.1	156	0
choc. fudge	2 T	4.0	110	1
choc. syrup, Hershey	2 T	0.4	73	1
marshmallow creme	3 T	0	158	0
milk choc. fudge	2 T	5.0	124	0
pineapple	3 T	0.2	146	0
strawberry	3 T	0.1	139	0
whipped topping				
aerosol	¼ cup	3.6	45	0
from mix	¼ cup	2.0	32	0
frzn, tub	¼ cup	4.8	59	0
"lite"	1 T	<1.0	8	0
whipping cream				
heavy, fluid	1 T	5.6	52	0
light, fluid	1 T	4.6	44	0
yogurt, frozen				
low fat	½ cup	1.0	120	0
nonfat	½ cup	0.2	100	0

Eggs

Item	Serving	Total Fat (g)	Calories	Fiber (g)
boiled-poached	1	5.6	79	0
fried w/½ t fat	1 large	7.8	104	0
omelet				
2 oz. cheese,				
3 egg	1	37.0	510	0
plain, 3 egg	1	21.3	271	0
Spanish, 2 egg	1	18.0	250	1
scrambled w/milk	1 large	8.0	99	0
substitute, frzn	¼ cup	0	30	0
white	1 large	0	16	0
yolk	1 large	5.6	63	0

Fats

Item	Serving	Total Fat (g)	Calories	Fiber (g)
bacon fat	1 T	14.0	126	0
beef, separable fat	1 oz.	23.3	216	0
butter				
solid	1 t	4.1	36	0
solid	1 T	12.3	108	0
whipped	1 t	3.1	28	0
Butter Buds, liquid	2 T	0	12	0
butter sprinkles	½ t	0	4	0
chicken fat, raw	1 T	12.8	115	0
cream				
light	1 T	2.9	29	0
medium (25% fat)	1 T	3.8	37	0
cream substitute				
liquid/frzn	½ fl. oz.	1.5	20	0
powdered	1 T	0.7	11	0
half & half	1 T	1.7	20	0
margarine				
liquid	1 t	4.0	36	0
reduced calorie,				
tub	1 t	2.0	18	0
solid (corn), stick	1 t	4.0	35	0
mayonnaise				
fat-free	1 T	0	12	0
reduced calorie	1 T	5.0	50	0
regular (soybean)	1 T	11.0	100	0
no-stick spray				
(Pam, etc.)	2-sec. spray	0.9	8	0
oil, all	1 T	14.0	120	0
pork fat (lard)	1 T	12.8	116	0
sandwich spread				
(Miracle Whip				
type)	1 T	7.0	69	0
shortening, vegetable	1 T	12.0	106	0
sour cream				
cultured	1 T	2.5	26	0
fat-free	1 T	0	8	0
half & half, cultured	1 T	1.8	20	0
imitation	1 T	2.7	30	0
"lite"	1 T	0.7	18	0

Fish (all baked/broiled w/o added fat unless otherwise noted)

Item	Serving	Total Fat (g)	Calories	Fiber (g)
anchovy, canned	3 fillets	1.1	25	0
bass				
freshwater	3½ oz.	4.7	145	0
saltwater, baked				
w/fat	3½ oz.	19.4	287	0
saltwater, black	3½ oz.	1.2	93	0
saltwater, striped	3½ oz.	2.5	105	0
bluefish				
cooked	3½ oz.	5.4	157	0
fried	3½ oz.	12.8	205	0
butterfish				
gulf	3½ oz.	2.9	95	0
northern	3½ oz.	10.2	184	0
northern, fried	3½ oz.	19.1	275	0
carp	3½ oz.	6.1	138	0
catfish	3½ oz.	3.1	103	0
catfish, breaded &				
fried	3½ oz.	13.2	226	NA
caviar, sturgeon,				
granular	1 round t	1.5	26	0

Item	Serving	Total Fat (g)	Calories	Fiber (g)
clams				
canned, solids & liquid	½ cup	0.7	85	0
canned, solids only	3 oz.	1.6	118	0
meat only	5 large	1.0	80	0
soft, raw	4 large	0.8	63	0
cod				
canned	3½ oz.	0.8	104	0
cooked	3½ oz.	0.8	104	0
dried, salted	3½ oz.	2.3	287	0
crab				
canned	½ cup	0.9	67	0
deviled	3½ oz.	10.1	217	0
fried	3½ oz.	18.0	273	0
crab, Alaska king	3½ oz.	1.5	96	0
crab cake	3½ oz.	10.8	178	0
crappie, white	3½ oz.	0.8	79	0
crayfish, freshwater	3½ oz.	1.4	113	0
cusk, steamed	3½ oz.	0.9	111	0
dolphinfish	3½ oz.	0.8	93	0
eel, American				
cooked	3½ oz.	18.3	260	0
smoked	3½ oz.	23.6	281	0
fillets, frzn				
batter dipped	2 pieces	25.8	447	0
light & crispy	2 pieces	15.9	301	0
fish cakes, frzn, fried	3½ oz.	14.0	242	2
flatfish	3½ oz.	0.8	79	0
flounder/sole	3½ oz.	0.5	68	0
gefilte fish	3½ oz.	2.2	82	1
grouper	3½ oz.	1.3	87	0
haddock				
cooked	3½ oz.	0.6	79	0
fried	3½ oz.	14.2	284	0
smoked/canned	3½ oz.	0.4	103	0
halibut	3½ oz.	1.2	100	0
herring				
canned or smoked	3½ oz.	13.6	208	0
cooked	3½ oz.	11.3	176	0
pickled	3½ oz.	15.1	223	0
Jack mackerel	3½ oz.	5.6	143	0
lake trout	3½ oz.	9.9	241	0
lobster, northern				
broiled w/fat	12 oz.	15.1	445	0
cooked	3½ oz.	0.6	97	0
mackerel				
Atlantic	3½ oz.	2.2	191	0
Pacific	3½ oz.	7.3	159	0
mussels				
canned	3½ oz.	4.5	163	0
meat only	3½ oz.	2.2	95	0
ocean perch				
cooked	3½ oz.	1.2	88	0
fried	3½ oz.	14.0	280	0
octopus	3½ oz.	2.1	163	0
oysters				
canned	3½ oz.	2.2	76	0
fried	3½ oz.	13.9	239	0
raw	5–8 medium	1.8	66	0
scalloped	6 medium	18.0	356	0
perch, freshwater,				
yellow	3½ oz.	0.9	91	0
pickerel	3½ oz.	0.5	84	0
pike				
blue	3½ oz.	0.9	90	0
northern	3½ oz.	1.1	88	0
walleye	3½ oz.	1.2	93	0
pollock, Atlantic	3½ oz.	1.0	91	0
pompano	3½ oz.	9.5	166	0
red snapper	3½ oz.	1.9	93	0
roughy, orange	3½ oz.	7.0	124	0
salmon				
Atlantic	3½ oz.	6.3	141	0
broiled/baked	3½ oz.	7.4	182	0
chinook, canned	3½ oz.	14.0	210	0
pink, canned	3½ oz.	5.1	118	0
smoked	3½ oz.	9.3	176	0
sardines				
Atlantic, in soy oil	2 sardines	2.8	50	0
Pacific	3½ oz.	8.6	160	0
scallops				
cooked	3½ oz.	1.2	81	0
frzn, fried	3½ oz.	10.5	194	0
steamed	3½ oz.	1.4	112	0
sea bass, white	3½ oz.	1.5	96	0
shrimp				
canned, dry pack	3½ oz.	1.6	116	0
canned, wet pack	½ cup	0.8	87	0
fried	3½ oz.	10.8	225	0
raw or boiled	3½ oz.	1.8	105	0
smelt, canned	4–5 medium	13.5	200	0
sole, fillet	3½ oz.	0.5	68	0
squid				
fried	3 oz.	6.4	149	0
raw	3 oz.	1.2	78	0
surimi	3½ oz.	0.9	98	0
sushi or sashimi	3½ oz.	4.9	144	0
swordfish	3½ oz.	4.0	118	0
trout				
brook	3½ oz.	2.1	101	0
rainbow	3½ oz.	11.4	195	0
tuna				
albacore, raw	3½ oz.	7.5	177	0
bluefin, raw	3½ oz.	4.1	145	0
canned, light in oil	3½ oz.	8.1	197	0
canned, light in water	3½ oz.	0.8	115	0
canned, white in oil	3½ oz.	8.0	185	0
canned, white in water	3½ oz.	2.4	135	0
yellowfin, raw	3½ oz.	3.0	133	0
white perch	3½ oz.	3.9	114	0
whiting	3½ oz.	1.7	114	0
yellowtail	3½ oz.	5.4	138	0

Fruit

Item	Serving	Total Fat (g)	Calories	Fiber (g)
apple				
dried	½ cup	0.1	155	5
whole w/peel	1 medium	0.4	81	4
applesauce,				
unsweetened	½ cup	0.1	53	2
apricots				
dried	5 halves	0.2	83	6
fresh	3 medium	0.4	51	2
avocado				
California	1 (6 oz.)	30.0	306	4
Florida	1 (11 oz.)	27.0	339	4
banana	1 medium	0.6	105	2
banana chips	½ cup	8.0	248	4
blackberries				
fresh	1 cup	0.6	74	7
frzn, unsweetened	1 cup	0.7	97	7
blueberries				
fresh	1 cup	0.6	82	5
frzn, unsweetened	1 cup	0.7	80	4
boysenberries, frzn,				
unsweetened	1 cup	0.4	66	6
breadfruit, fresh	¼ small	0.2	99	3
cantaloupe	1 cup	0.4	57	3
cherries				
maraschino	¼ cup	0.2	66	1
sour, canned in				
heavy syrup	½ cup	0.1	116	1
sweet	½ cup	0.7	49	2
cranberries, fresh	1 cup	0.2	46	4
cranberry-orange relish	½ cup	0.9	246	3
cranberry sauce	½ cup	0.2	209	1
dates, whole, dried	½ cup	0.4	228	8
figs				
canned	3 figs	0.1	75	9
dried, uncooked	10 figs	1.1	254	10
fresh	1 medium	0.2	37	2
fruit cocktail, canned				
w/juice	1 cup	0.3	112	5
fruit roll-up	1	0	50	0
grapefruit	½ medium	0.1	39	1
grapes, Thompson				
seedless	½ cup	0.1	94	1
guava, fresh	1 medium	0.5	45	7
honeydew melon,				
fresh	¼ small	0.1	46	1
kiwi, fresh	1 medium	0.3	46	2
kumquat, fresh	1 medium	0	12	1
lemon, fresh	1 medium	0.2	17	1
lime, fresh	1 medium	0.1	20	1
mandarin oranges,				
canned w/juice	½ cup	0	46	4
mango, fresh	1 medium	0.6	135	4
melon balls, frzn	1 cup	0.4	55	2
mixed fruit				
dried	½ cup	0.5	243	6
frzn, sweetened	1 cup	0.5	245	2
mulberries, fresh	1 cup	0.6	61	3

Item	Serving	Total Fat (g)	Calories	Fiber (g)
nectarine, fresh	1 medium	0.6	67	2
orange				
navel, fresh	1 medium	0.1	65	4
Valencia, fresh	1 medium	0.4	59	4
papaya, fresh	1 medium	0.4	117	3
passionfruit, purple,				
fresh	1 medium	0.1	18	3
peach				
canned, water pack	1 cup	0.1	58	4
canned in heavy				
syrup	1 cup	0.3	190	4
canned in light syrup	1 cup	0.1	136	4
fresh	1 medium	0.1	37	1
frzn, sweetened	1 cup	0.3	235	4
pear				
canned in heavy				
syrup	1 cup	0.3	188	6
canned in light syrup	1 cup	0.1	144	6
fresh	1 medium	0.7	98	5
persimmon, fresh	1 medium	0.1	32	3
pineapple pieces				
canned, unsweetened	1 cup	0.2	150	2
fresh	1 cup	0.7	77	3
plantain, cooked,				
sliced	1 cup	0.3	179	1
plum				
canned in heavy				
syrup	½ cup	0.1	119	4
fresh	1 medium	0.4	36	3
pomegranate, fresh	1 medium	0.5	104	2
prickly pear, fresh	1 medium	0.5	42	3
prunes, dried, cooked	½ cup	0.2	113	10
raisins				
dark seedless	¼ cup	0.2	112	3
golden seedless	¼ cup	0.2	113	3
raspberries				
fresh	1 cup	0.7	61	6
frzn, sweetened	1 cup	0.4	256	12
rhubarb, diced,				
unsweetened	1 cup	0.2	26	6
star fruit/carambola	1 medium	0.4	42	2
strawberries				
fresh	1 cup	0.6	45	3
frzn, sweetened	1 cup	0.3	245	3
frzn, unsweetened	1 cup	0.2	52	3
sugar apples, fresh	1 medium	0.5	146	4
tangelo, fresh	1 medium	0.1	39	3
tangerine, fresh	1 medium	0.2	37	3
watermelon, fresh	1 cup	0.5	50	1

Fruit Juices and Nectars

Item	Serving	Total Fat (g)	Calories	Fiber (g)
apple juice	1 cup	0.3	116	1
apricot nectar	1 cup	0.2	141	1
carrot juice	1 cup	0.4	97	1
cranberry-apple juice	1 cup	0.2	160	1
cranberry juice cocktail				
low cal	1 cup	0	45	0
regular	1 cup	0.1	144	0

Item	Serving	Total Fat (g)	Calories	Fiber (g)
grape juice	1 cup	0.2	128	1
grapefruit juice	1 cup	0.2	93	0
lemon juice	2 T	0	5	0
lime juice	2 T	0	6	0
orange-grapefruit juice	1 cup	0.2	107	1
orange juice	1 cup	0.5	111	1
peach juice or nectar	1 cup	0.1	134	1
pear juice or nectar	1 cup	0	149	1
pineapple juice	1 cup	0.2	139	1
pineapple-orange juice	1 cup	0.1	133	1
prune juice	1 cup	0.1	181	1
tomato juice	1 cup	0.2	43	2
V8 juice	1 cup	0.1	49	2

Gravies, Sauces, and Dips

Item	Serving	Total Fat (g)	Calories	Fiber (g)
au jus, mix	½ cup	0.3	24	0
barbecue sauce	1 T	0.3	12	0
bèarnaise sauce, mix	¼ pkg.	25.6	263	0
brown gravy				
from mix	½ cup	0.9	38	0
hmde	¼ cup	14.0	164	0
catsup, tomato	1 T	0.1	16	0
chicken gravy				
canned	½ can	6.5	95	0
from mix	½ cup	0.9	41	0
giblet from can	¼ cup	1.5	29	0
chili sauce	1 T	0	16	0
guacamole dip	1 oz.	4.0	50	0
hollandaise sauce	¼ cup	18.0	170	0
home-style gravy,				
from mix	¼ cup	0.5	25	0
mushroom gravy				
canned	½ can	4.0	75	0
from mix	½ cup	0.4	35	0
mushroom sauce,				
from mix	¼ pkg	3.2	71	0
mustard				
brown	1 T	0.9	15	0
yellow	1 T	0.6	12	0
onion dip	2 T	4.0	45	0
onion gravy, from				
mix	½ cup	0.4	39	0
pesto sauce,				
commercial	1 oz.	14.6	155	0
picante sauce	6 T	0	36	1
pork gravy, from mix	½ cup	0.9	38	0
sour-cream sauce	¼ cup	7.6	128	0
soy sauce	1 T	0	11	0
soy sauce, reduced				
sodium	1 T	0	11	0
spaghetti sauce				
"healthy"/"lite"				
varieties	½ cup	1.0	60	1
hmde, w/reg.				
ground beef	½ cup	18.7	243	1
meat flavor, jar	½ cup	6.0	100	1
meatless, jar	½ cup	2.0	70	NA
mushroom, jar	½ cup	2.0	70	NA

Item	Serving	Total Fat (g)	Calories	Fiber (g)
steak sauce				
A-1	1 T	0	12	0
others	1 T	0	18	0
tabasco sauce	1 t	0	1	0
taco sauce	1 T	0	5	0
tartar sauce	1 T	7.7	70	0
teriyaki sauce	1 T	0	15	0
turkey gravy				
canned	½ can	3.1	76	0
from mix	½ cup	0.9	43	0
white sauce	2 T	3.4	60	0
Worcestershire sauce	1 T	0	10	0

Meats (all cooked w/o added fat unless otherwise noted)

Item	Serving	Total Fat (g)	Calories	Fiber (g)
beef, extra lean, <5% fat by weight (cooked)				
Healthy Choice lean ground beef	3½ oz.	3.5	114	0
round, eye of, lean	3½ oz.	3.5	155	0
beef, lean, 5–10% fat by weight (cooked)				
flank steak, fat trimmed	3½ oz.	8.0	193	0
round				
bottom, lean	3½ oz.	9.4	207	0
top, lean	3½ oz.	6.4	211	0
sirloin tip, lean, roasted	3½ oz.	9.4	207	0
tenderloin, lean, broiled	3½ oz.	11.1	219	0
top sirloin, lean, broiled	3½ oz.	7.9	201	0
beef, regular, 11–17.4% fat by weight (cooked)				
chuck, separable lean	3½ oz.	15.2	268	0
club steak, lean	3½ oz.	12.9	240	0
hamburger				
extra lean	3 oz.	13.9	253	0
lean	3 oz.	15.7	268	0
sirloin tips, roasted	3½ oz.	15.2	264	0
stew meat, round, raw	4 oz.	15.3	294	0
tenderloin, marbled	3½ oz.	15.2	264	0
beef, high fat, 17.5–27.4% fat by weight (cooked)				
chuck, ground	3½ oz.	23.9	327	0
hamburger, regular	3 oz.	19.6	286	0
meatballs	1 oz.	5.5	78	0
porterhouse steak, lean & marbled	3½ oz.	19.6	286	0
rib steak	3½ oz.	14.7	286	0
rump, pot-roasted	3½ oz.	19.6	286	0
short ribs, lean	3½ oz.	19.6	286	0

Item	Serving	Total Fat (g)	Calories	Fiber (g)
sirloin, broiled	3½ oz.	18.7	278	0
sirloin, ground	3½ oz.	26.5	354	0
T-bone, broiled	3½ oz.	26.5	354	0
beef, highest fat, ≥27.5% fat by weight (cooked)				
brisket, lean & marbled	3½ oz.	30.0	367	0
chuck, stew meat	3½ oz.	30.0	367	0
corned, medium fat	3½ oz.	30.2	372	0
ribeye steak, marbled	3½ oz.	38.8	440	0
rib roast	3½ oz.	30.0	367	0
short ribs	3½ oz.	31.7	382	0
steak, chicken fried	3½ oz.	30.0	389	0
lamb				
blade chop				
lean	1 chop	6.4	128	0
lean & marbled	3½ oz.	26.1	380	0
leg				
lean	3½ oz.	8.1	180	0
lean & marbled	3½ oz.	14.5	242	0
loin chop				
lean	3½ oz.	8.1	180	0
lean & marbled	3½ oz.	22.5	302	0
rib chop				
lean	3½ oz.	8.1	180	0
lean & marbled	3½ oz.	21.2	292	0
shoulder				
lean	3½ oz.	9.9	248	0
lean & marbled	3½ oz.	27.0	430	0
miscellaneous meats				
bacon substitute (breakfast strip)	2 strips	4.8	50	0
beefalo	3½ oz.	6.3	188	0
venison, roasted	3½ oz.	2.5	157	0
organ meats				
brains, all kinds, raw	3 oz.	7.4	106	0
heart, beef, lean, braised	3½ oz.	5.6	175	0
kidney, beef, braised	3½ oz.	3.4	144	0
liver				
beef, braised	3½ oz.	4.9	161	0
beef, pan fried	3½ oz.	8.0	217	0
calf, braised	3½ oz.	6.9	165	0
calf, pan fried	3½ oz.	11.4	245	0
pork				
bacon				
cured, broiled	1 slice	3.1	35	0
cured, raw	1 oz.	11.0	115	0
bacon bits	1 T	1.0	20	0
blade				
lean	3½ oz.	9.6	219	0
lean & marbled	3½ oz.	18.0	290	0
Boston butt				
lean	3½ oz.	14.2	304	0
lean & marbled	3½ oz.	28.0	348	0
Canadian bacon, broiled	1 oz.	1.8	43	0

Item	Serving	Total Fat (g)	Calories	Fiber (g)
ham				
cured, butt, lean	3½ oz.	4.5	159	0
cured, butt, lean & marbled	3½ oz.	13.0	246	0
cured, canned	3 oz.	5.0	120	0
cured, shank, lean	3½ oz.	6.3	164	0
cured, shank, lean & marbled	2 slices	13.8	255	0
fresh, lean	3½ oz.	6.4	222	0
fresh, lean, marbled & fat	3½ oz.	18.3	306	0
smoked	3½ oz.	7.0	140	0
loin chop				
lean	1 chop	7.7	170	0
lean & fat	1 chop	22.5	314	0
picnic				
cured, lean	3½ oz.	9.9	211	0
fresh, lean	3½ oz.	7.4	150	0
shoulder, lean	2 slices	5.4	162	0
shoulder, marbled	2 slices	14.3	234	0
rib chop, trimmed	3½ oz.	9.9	209	0
rib roast, trimmed	3½ oz.	10.0	204	0
sausage				
brown and serve	1 oz.	9.4	105	0
patty	1	8.4	100	0
regular link	½ oz.	4.7	52	0
sirloin, lean, roasted	3½ oz.	10.2	207	0
spareribs, roasted	6 medium	35.0	396	0
tenderloin, lean, roast	3½ oz.	4.8	155	0
top loin chop, trimmed	3½ oz.	7.7	193	0
top loin roast, trimmed	3½ oz.	7.5	187	0
processed meats				
bacon substitute (breakfast strips)	2 strips	4.8	50	0
beef breakfast strips	2 strips	7.0	100	0
bologna, beef/beef & pork	1 oz.	8.3	90	0
bratwurst				
pork	2-oz. link	22.0	256	0
pork & beef	2-oz. link	19.5	226	0
braunshweiger (pork liver sausage)	1 oz.	5.8	65	0
corn dog	1	20.0	330	0
ham, chopped	1 oz.	2.3	55	0
hot dog/frank				
beef	1	13.2	145	0
chicken	1	8.8	116	0
97% fat free varieties	1	1.6	55	0
turkey	1	8.1	102	0
kielbasa (Polish sausage)	1 oz.	8.3	80	0
knockwurst/ knackwurst	2-oz. link	18.9	209	0
pepperoni	1 oz.	13.0	140	0
salami				
cooked	1 oz.	10.0	116	0
dry/hard	1 oz.	10.0	120	0

Item	Serving	Total Fat (g)	Calories	Fiber (g)
sausage				
Italian	2-oz. link	17.2	216	0
90% fat free				
varieties	1 oz.	2.3	43	0
Polish	1-oz. link	8.1	92	0
smoked	2-oz. link	20.0	229	0
Vienna	1 sausage	4.0	45	0
Spam	1 oz.	8.0	86	0
turkey breast	1 oz.	0.8	31	0
turkey ham	1 oz.	1.5	36	0
turkey loaf	1 oz.	2.7	43	0
turkey pastrami	1 oz.	1.8	40	0
turkey roll	1 oz.	4.5	72	0
turkey salami	1 oz.	3.7	55	0
veal				
arm steak				
lean	3½ oz.	4.8	180	0
lean & fat	3½ oz.	19.0	298	0
blade				
lean	3½ oz.	8.4	228	0
lean & fat	3½ oz.	16.6	276	0
breast, stewed	3½ oz.	18.6	256	0
chuck, med. fat,				
braised	3½ oz.	12.8	235	0
cutlet				
breaded	3½ oz.	15.0	319	0
round, lean	3½ oz.	12.8	194	0
round, lean & fat	3½ oz.	15.0	277	0
flank, med. fat,				
stewed	3½ oz.	32.0	390	0
foreshank, med. fat,				
stewed	3½ oz.	10.4	216	0
loin, med. fat,				
broiled	3½ oz.	13.4	234	0
loin chop				
lean	1 chop	4.8	149	0
lean & fat	3½ oz.	13.3	250	0
plate, med. fat,				
stewed	3½ oz.	21.2	303	0
rib chop				
lean	1 chop	4.6	125	0
lean & fat	1 chop	18.4	264	0
rump, marbled,				
roasted	3½ oz.	11.0	225	0
sirloin				
lean, roasted	3½ oz.	3.4	175	0
marbled, roasted	3½ oz.	6.5	181	0
sirloin steak				
lean	3½ oz.	6.0	204	0
lean & fat	3½ oz.	20.4	305	0

Milk and Yogurt

Item	Serving	Total Fat (g)	Calories	Fiber (g)
buttermilk				
1% fat	1 cup	2.2	99	0
dry	1 T	0.4	25	0
choc. milk				
2% fat	1 cup	5.0	179	0
whole	1 cup	8.5	250	0

Item	Serving	Total Fat (g)	Calories	Fiber (g)
condensed milk,				
sweetened	½ cup	13.3	491	0
evaporated milk				
skim	½ cup	0.4	100	0
whole	½ cup	9.5	169	0
hot cocoa				
low cal. mix				
w/water	1 cup	0.8	50	0
mix w/water	1 cup	3.0	110	0
w/skim milk	1 cup	2.0	158	0
w/whole milk	1 cup	9.1	218	0
low-fat milk				
½% fat	1 cup	1.0	90	0
1% fat	1 cup	2.6	102	0
1.5% fat/acidophilus	1 cup	4.0	110	0
2% fat	1 cup	4.7	121	0
milkshake				
choc., thick	1 cup	6.1	267	1
soft serve	1 cup	7.0	218	1
vanilla, thick	1 cup	6.9	255	0
skim milk				
liquid	1 cup	0.4	86	0
nonfat dry powder	¼ cup	0.2	109	0
whole milk				
3.5% fat	1 cup	8.2	150	0
dry powder	¼ cup	8.6	159	0
yogurt				
coffee/vanilla, low fat	1 cup	2.8	194	0
frzn, low fat	½ cup	3.0	115	0
frzn, nonfat	½ cup	0.2	81	0
fruit flavored, low fat	1 cup	2.6	225	0
plain				
low fat	1 cup	3.5	144	0
skim (nonfat)	1 cup	0.4	127	0
whole milk	1 cup	7.4	139	0

Miscellaneous

Item	Serving	Total Fat (g)	Calories	Fiber (g)
baking powder	1 t	0	3	0
baking soda	1 t	0	0	0
bouillon cube, beef or				
chicken	1	0.2	9	0
chewing gum	1 stick	0	10	0
choc., baking	1 oz.	15.7	148	1
cocoa, dry	⅓ cup	3.6	115	2
honey	1 T	0	64	0
horseradish, prepared	1 t	0	2	0
jam, all varieties	1 T	0	54	0
jelly, all varieties	1 T	0	49	0
marmalade, citrus	1 T	0	51	0
meat tenderizer	1 t	0	2	0
molasses	1 T	0	50	0
olives				
black	2 large	4.0	37	1
Greek	3 medium	7.1	67	1
green	2 medium	1.6	15	0
pickle relish				
chow chow	1 oz.	0.4	8	0
sweet	1 T	0.1	21	0

Item	Serving	Total Fat (g)	Calories	Fiber (g)
pickles				
bread & butter	4 slices	0.1	18	0
dill or sour	1 large	0.1	12	1
Kosher	1 oz.	0.1	7	0
sweet	1 oz.	0.4	146	0
salt	1 t	0	0	0
Shake & Bake, Gen.				
Foods	¼ pkg.	2.0	80	0
spices/seasonings	1 t	0.2	5	0
sugar, all varieties	1 T	0	46	0
sugar substitutes	1 packet	0	4	0
syrup, all varieties	1 T	0	60	0
vinegar	1 T	0	2	0
yeast	1 T	0	23	0

Nuts and Seeds

Item	Serving	Total Fat (g)	Calories	Fiber (g)
almonds	12–15	9.3	104	1
Brazil nuts	4 medium	11.5	114	1
cashews, roasted	6–8	7.8	94	2
chestnuts, fresh	3 small	0.8	66	4
coconut, dried,				
shredded	⅓ cup	9.2	135	1
hazelnuts (filberts)	10–12	10.6	106	1
macadamia nuts,				
roasted	6 medium	12.3	117	1
mixed nuts				
w/peanuts	8–12	10.0	109	2
w/o peanuts	2 T	10.1	110	2
peanut butter, creamy				
or chunky	1 T	8.0	94	1
peanuts				
chopped	2 T	8.9	104	2
honey roasted	2 T	8.9	112	2
in shell	1 cup	17.7	209	3
pecans	2 T	9.1	90	1
pine nuts (pignolia)	2 T	9.1	85	2
pistachios	2 T	7.7	92	1
poppy seeds	1 T	3.8	44	1
pumpkin seeds	2 T	7.9	93	1
sesame nut mix	2 T	5.1	65	1
sesame seeds	2 T	8.8	94	1
sunflower seeds	2 T	8.9	102	1
trail mix w/seeds,				
nuts, carob	2 T	5.1	87	1
walnuts	2 T	7.7	80	1

Pasta, Noodles, and Rice (all measurements after cooking unless otherwise noted; 2 oz. uncooked pasta = ~1 cup cooked)

Item	Serving	Total Fat (g)	Calories	Fiber (g)
macaroni				
semolina	1 cup	0.7	210	1
whole wheat	1 cup	2.0	210	5
noodles				
Alfredo	1 cup	29.7	462	3
almondine, from mix	¼ pkg.	12.0	240	1
cellophane, fried	1 cup	4.2	141	0
chow mein, canned	½ cup	8.0	150	0
egg	1 cup	2.4	212	1
manicotti	1 cup	1.0	210	1
ramen, all varieties	1 cup	8.0	190	1
rice	1 cup	0.3	140	1
romanoff	1 cup	23.0	372	3
rice				
brown	½ cup	0.6	116	2
fried	½ cup	7.2	181	1
long grain & wild	½ cup	2.1	120	2
pilaf	½ cup	7.0	170	1
Spanish style	½ cup	2.1	106	1
white	½ cup	1.2	111	0
spaghetti, enriched	1 cup	1.0	210	1

Poultry

Item	Serving	Total Fat (g)	Calories	Fiber (g)
chicken				
breast				
w/skin, fried	½ breast	10.7	236	0
w/o skin, fried	½ breast	6.1	179	0
w/skin, roasted	½ breast	7.6	193	0
w/o skin, roasted	½ breast	3.1	142	0
fryers				
w/skin, batter				
dipped, fried	3½ oz.	17.4	289	0
w/o skin, fried	3½ oz.	11.1	237	0
w/skin, roasted	3½ oz.	13.6	239	0
w/o skin, roasted	3½ oz.	7.4	190	0
giblets, fried	3½ oz.	13.5	277	0
leg				
w/skin, fried	1 leg	8.7	120	0
w/skin, roasted	1 leg	5.8	112	0
w/o skin, roasted	1 leg	2.5	76	0
roll, light meat	3½ oz.	7.4	159	0
stewers				
w/skin	3½ oz.	18.9	285	0
w/o skin	3½ oz.	11.9	237	0
thigh				
w/skin, fried	1 thigh	11.3	180	0
w/skin, roasted	1 thigh	9.6	153	0
w/o skin, roasted	1 thigh	5.7	109	0
wing				
w/skin, fried	1 wing	9.1	121	0
w/skin, roasted	1 wing	6.6	99	0
duck				
w/skin, roasted	3½ oz.	28.4	337	0
w/o skin, roasted	3½ oz.	11.2	201	0
turkey				
breast				
barbecued,				
Louis Rich	3½ oz.	3.2	118	0
oven roasted,				
Louis Rich	3½ oz.	3.2	111	0
smoked, Louis Rich	3½ oz.	3.7	118	0
dark meat				
w/skin, roasted	3½ oz.	11.5	221	0
w/o skin, roasted	3½ oz.	7.2	187	0
ground	3½ oz.	13.3	219	0
ham, cured	3½ oz.	5.1	128	0

Item	Serving	Total Fat (g)	Calories	Fiber (g)
light meat				
w/skin, roasted	3½ oz.	8.3	197	0
w/o skin, roasted	3½ oz.	3.2	157	0
roll, light meat	3½ oz.	7.2	147	0
sausage, cooked	1 oz.	3.4	50	0
sliced w/gravy, frzn	5 oz.	3.7	95	0

Salad Dressings

Item	Serving	Total Fat (g)	Calories	Fiber (g)
blue cheese				
fat free	1 T	0	10	0
low cal	1 T	1.9	27	0
regular	1 T	8.0	77	0
buttermilk, from mix	1 T	5.8	58	0
Caesar	1 T	7.0	70	0
French				
creamy	1 T	6.9	70	0
fat free	1 T	0	18	0
low cal	1 T	0.9	22	0
regular	1 T	6.4	67	0
garlic, from mix	1 T	9.2	85	0
Green Goddess				
low cal	1 T	2.0	27	0
regular	1 T	7.0	68	0
honey mustard	1 T	6.6	89	0
Italian				
creamy	1 T	5.5	54	0
fat free	1 T	0	6	0
low cal	1 T	1.5	16	0
regular zesty, from mix	1 T	9.2	85	0
Kraft, free	1 T	0	20	0
Kraft, reduced cal	1 T	1.0	25	0
mayonnaise type				
low cal	1 T	1.8	19	0
regular	1 T	4.9	57	0
oil & vinegar	1 T	7.5	69	0
ranch style, prep. w/mayo	1 T	6.0	58	0
Russian				
low cal	1 T	0.7	24	0
regular	1 T	7.8	76	0
sesame seed	1 T	6.9	68	0
sweet & sour	1 T	0.9	29	0
Thousand Island				
fat free	1 T	0	20	0
low cal	1 T	1.6	24	0
regular	1 T	5.6	59	0

Snack Foods

Item	Serving	Total Fat (g)	Calories	Fiber (g)
bagel chips or crisps	1 oz.	4.0	130	1
Cheese Puffs, Cheetos	1 oz.	10.0	160	0
corn chips, Frito's				
barbecue	1 oz.	9.0	150	0
regular	1 oz.	10.0	160	0
Cracker Jack	1 oz.	3.0	120	1
party mix (cereal, pretzels, nuts)	1 cup	23.0	312	3

Item	Serving	Total Fat (g)	Calories	Fiber (g)
popcorn				
air popped	1 cup	0.3	31	1
caramel	1 cup	4.5	150	1
microwave, "lite"	1 cup	1.0	27	1
microwave, plain	1 cup	3.0	47	1
microwave, w/butter	1 cup	4.5	61	1
popped w/oil	1 cup	3.1	55	1
potato chips				
individually	10 chips	8.0	113	0
by weight	1 oz.	11.2	159	1
barbecue flavor	1 oz.	9.5	149	1
light, Pringles	1 oz.	8.0	150	0
regular, Pringles	1 oz.	12.0	170	0
pretzels	1 oz.	1.0	110	0
rice cakes	1	0	35	0
tortilla chips				
Doritos	1 oz.	6.6	139	0
no oil, baked	1 oz.	1.5	110	0
Tostitos	1 oz.	7.8	145	0

Soups

Item	Serving	Total Fat (g)	Calories	Fiber (g)
bean				
w/bacon	1 cup	5.9	173	4
w/franks	1 cup	7.0	187	3
w/ham	1 cup	8.5	231	3
w/o meat	1 cup	3.0	142	5
beef				
broth	1 cup	0.5	33	0
chunky	1 cup	5.1	171	2
beef barley	1 cup	1.1	72	1
beef noodle	1 cup	3.1	84	1
black bean	1 cup	1.5	116	2
broccoli, creamy w/water	1 cup	2.8	69	1
canned vegetable type, w/o meat	1 cup	1.6	59	1
cheese w/milk	1 cup	14.6	230	0
chicken				
chunky	1 cup	6.6	178	2
cream of, w/milk	1 cup	11.5	191	0
cream of, w/water	1 cup	7.4	116	0
chicken & wild rice	1 cup	2.3	76	1
chicken/beef noodle or veg.	1 cup	3.1	83	1
chicken gumbo	1 cup	1.4	56	1
chicken mushroom	1 cup	9.2	132	1
chicken noodle				
chunky	1 cup	5.2	149	2
w/water	1 cup	2.5	75	0
chicken vegetable				
chunky	1 cup	4.8	167	2
w/water	1 cup	2.8	74	1
chicken w/noodles, chunky	1 cup	5.0	180	2
chicken w/rice				
chunky	1 cup	3.2	127	2
w/water	1 cup	1.9	60	1

Item	Serving	Total Fat (g)	Calories	Fiber (g)
clam chowder				
Manhattan chunky	1 cup	3.4	133	1
New England	1 cup	6.6	163	1
consommé w/gelatin	1 cup	0	29	0
crab	1 cup	1.5	76	1
dehydrated				
asparagus, cream of	1 cup	1.7	59	0
bean w/bacon	1 cup	3.5	105	2
beef broth cube	1 cube	0.3	6	0
beef noodle	1 cup	0.8	41	0
cauliflower	1 cup	1.7	68	0
chicken, cream of	1 cup	5.3	107	1
chicken broth cube	1 cube	0.2	9	0
chicken noodle	1 cup	1.2	53	0
chicken rice	1 cup	1.4	60	0
clam chowder				
Manhattan	1 cup	1.6	65	1
New England	1 cup	3.7	95	0
minestrone	1 cup	1.7	79	0
mushroom	1 cup	4.9	96	0
onion				
dry mix	1 pkg.	2.3	115	1
prepared	1 cup	0.6	28	0
tomato	1 cup	2.4	102	0
vegetable beef	1 cup	1.1	53	0
gazpacho	1 cup	0.2	40	2
hmde or restaurant style				
cauliflower, cream of,				
w/whole milk	1 cup	9.7	165	1
celery, cream of,				
w/whole milk	1 cup	10.6	165	1
chicken broth	1 cup	1.4	38	0
clam chowder				
Manhattan	1 cup	2.2	76	2
New England	1 cup	14.0	271	1
corn chowder,				
traditional	1 cup	12.0	251	3
fish chowder,				
w/whole milk	1 cup	13.5	285	1
gazpacho, traditional	1 cup	7.0	100	2
onion, French w/o				
cheese	1 cup	5.8	114	0
oyster stew,				
w/whole milk	1 cup	17.7	268	0
seafood gumbo	1 cup	3.9	155	3
lentil	1 cup	1.0	161	3
minestrone				
chunky	1 cup	2.8	127	2
w/water	1 cup	2.5	83	1
mushroom, cream of				
condensed	1 can	23.1	313	1
w/milk	1 cup	13.6	203	1
w/water	1 cup	9.0	129	1
mushroom w/beef stock	1 cup	4.0	85	1
onion	1 cup	1.7	57	1
oyster stew, w/water	1 cup	3.8	59	1
pea				
green, w/water	1 cup	2.9	164	2
split	1 cup	0.6	58	1
split w/ham	1 cup	4.4	189	1
potato, cream of,				
w/milk	1 cup	7.4	157	2
shrimp, cream of,				
w/milk	1 cup	9.3	165	1
tomato				
w/milk	1 cup	6.0	160	1
w/water	1 cup	1.9	86	0.5
tomato beef w/noodle	1 cup	4.3	140	1
tomato rice	1 cup	2.7	120	1
turkey, chunky	1 cup	4.4	136	2
turkey noodle	1 cup	2.0	69	1
turkey vegetable	1 cup	3.0	74	1
vegetable, chunky	1 cup	3.7	122	2
vegetable w/beef,				
chunky	1 cup	3.0	134	2
vegetable				
w/beef broth	1 cup	1.9	80	1
vegetarian vegetable	1 cup	1.2	73	1
wonton	1 cup	1.0	40	1

Vegetables

Item	Serving	Total Fat (g)	Calories	Fiber (g)
alfalfa sprouts, raw	½ cup	0.1	5	0
artichoke, boiled	1 medium	0.2	53	3
artichoke hearts,				
boiled	½ cup	0.1	37	3
asparagus, cooked	½ cup	0.3	22	2
avocado				
California	1 (6 oz.)	30.0	306	4
Florida	1 (11 oz.)	27.0	339	4
bamboo shoots, raw	½ cup	0.2	21	2
beans				
all types, cooked				
w/o fat	½ cup	0.4	143	9
baked, brown sugar				
& molasses	½ cup	1.5	132	4
baked, vegetarian	½ cup	0.6	118	5
baked w/pork &				
tomato sauce	½ cup	1.3	123	5
homestyle, canned	½ cup	1.6	132	5
beets, pickled	½ cup	0.1	75	4
black-eyed peas				
(cowpeas), cooked	½ cup	0.6	100	2
broccoli				
cooked	½ cup	0.3	22	7
frzn, chopped,				
cooked	½ cup	0.1	25	2
frzn in butter sauce	½ cup	2.3	51	2
frzn w/cheese sauce	½ cup	6.2	116	1
raw	½ cup	0.2	12	1
brussels sprouts,				
cooked	½ cup	0.4	30	2
butter beans, canned	½ cup	0.4	76	4
cabbage				
Chinese, raw	1 cup	0.2	10	2
green, cooked	½ cup	0.1	16	2
red, raw, shredded	½ cup	0.1	10	2

Item	Serving	Total Fat (g)	Calories	Fiber (g)
carrot				
cooked	½ cup	0.1	35	2
raw	1 large	0.1	31	2
cauliflower				
cooked	1 cup	0.2	30	3
frzn w/cheese sauce	½ cup	6.1	114	2
raw	1 cup	0.1	12	4
celery				
cooked	½ cup	0.1	13	1
raw	1 stalk	0.1	6	1
chard, cooked	½ cup	0.1	18	2
chiles, green	¼ cup	0	10	0
Chinese-style				
vegetables, frzn	½ cup	4.0	74	3
chives, raw, chopped	1 T	0	1	0
collard greens,				
cooked	½ cup	0.1	13	2
corn				
corn on the cob	1 medium	1.0	120	4
cream style, canned	½ cup	0.5	93	4
frzn, cooked	½ cup	0.1	67	4
frzn w/butter sauce	½ cup	2.2	110	4
whole kernel,				
cooked	½ cup	1.1	89	5
cucumber				
w/skin	½ medium	0.2	20	1
w/o skin, sliced	½ cup	0.1	7	0
dandelion greens,				
cooked	½ cup	0.3	17	2
eggplant, cooked	½ cup	0.1	13	2
endive lettuce	1 cup	0.2	8	1
garbanzo beans (chick				
peas), cooked	½ cup	2.1	135	5
green beans				
french style, cooked	½ cup	0.2	26	2
snap, cooked	½ cup	0.2	22	2
hominy, white or				
yellow, cooked	1 cup	0.7	138	3
Italian-style vegetables,				
frzn	½ cup	5.5	102	2
kale, cooked	½ cup	0.3	21	2
kidney beans, red,				
cooked	½ cup	0.5	112	8
leeks, chopped, raw	¼ cup	0.1	16	1
lentils, cooked	½ cup	0.4	116	8
lettuce, leaf	1 cup	0.2	10	1
lima beans, cooked	½ cup	0.4	108	5
miso (soybean product)	½ cup	8.4	284	4
mushrooms				
canned	½ cup	0.2	19	1
fried/sautéed	4 medium	7.4	78	1
raw	½ cup	0.2	9	1
mustard greens,				
cooked	½ cup	0.2	11	2
okra, cooked	½ cup	0.1	25	3
onions				
canned, french-fried	1 oz.	15.0	175	0
chopped, raw	½ cup	0.1	30	1

Item	Serving	Total Fat (g)	Calories	Fiber (g)
parsley, chopped,				
raw	¼ cup	0.1	5	0
parsnips, cooked	½ cup	0.2	63	3
peas, green,				
cooked	½ cup	0.2	67	4
pepper, bell, chopped,				
raw	½ cup	0.1	13	2
pimientos, canned	1 oz.	0	10	0
potato				
au gratin				
from mix	½ cup	6.0	140	2
hmde	½ cup	9.3	160	1
baked w/skin	1 medium	0.2	220	4
boiled w/o skin	½ cup	0.1	116	2
french fries				
frzn	10 pieces	4.4	111	2
hmde	10 pieces	8.3	158	1
hash browns	½ cup	10.9	163	2
knishes	1	3.2	73	1
mashed				
from flakes, w/milk				
& marg.	½ cup	6.0	130	1
w/milk & marg.	½ cup	4.4	111	1
pan fried, O'Brien	½ cup	15.0	231	3
potato pancakes	1 cake	12.6	237	1
potato puffs, frzn,				
prep. w/oil	½ cup	11.6	183	3
scalloped				
from mix	1 serving	5.9	127	1
hmde	½ cup	4.8	105	1
w/cheese	½ cup	9.7	177	1
twice-baked potato,				
w/cheese	1 medium	9.9	180	1
pumpkin, canned	½ cup	0.3	41	4
radish, raw	10	0.2	7	1
rhubarb, raw	1 cup	0.2	29	2
sauerkraut, canned	½ cup	0.2	22	4
scallions, raw	5 medium	0.2	60	4
soybeans, mature,				
cooked	½ cup	7.7	149	4
spinach				
cooked	½ cup	0.2	21	3
creamed	½ cup	5.1	79	3
raw	1 cup	0.2	12	3
squash				
acorn				
baked	½ cup	0.1	57	4
mashed w/o fat	½ cup	0.1	41	3
butternut, cooked	½ cup	0.1	41	4
summer				
cooked	½ cup	0.3	18	2
raw, sliced	½ cup	0.1	13	1
winter, cooked	½ cup	0.6	39	4
succotash, cooked	½ cup	0.8	111	3
sweet potato				
baked	1 small	0.1	118	7
candied	½ cup	3.4	144	5
mashed w/o fat	½ cup	0.5	172	5

Item	Serving	Total Fat (g)	Calories	Fiber (g)
tempeh (soybean product)	½ cup	6.4	165	1
tofu (soybean curd), raw, firm	4 oz.	4.0	90	1
tomato				
boiled	½ cup	0.5	32	1
raw	1 medium	0.4	26	1
stewed	½ cup	0.2	34	1
tomato paste, canned	½ cup	1.2	110	4
turnip greens, cooked	½ cup	0.2	15	2
turnips, cooked	½ cup	0.1	14	2
water chestnuts, canned, sliced	½ cup	0	35	1
watercress, raw	½ cup	0	2	0
wax beans, canned	½ cup	0.2	25	2
yam, boiled/baked	½ cup	0.1	79	3
zucchini, cooked	½ cup	0.1	14	2
Vegetable Salads				
Caesar salad w/o anchovies	1 cup	7.2	80	1
carrot-raisin salad	½ cup	5.8	153	4
chef salad w/o dressing	1 cup	4.2	65	1
coleslaw				
w/mayo-type dressing	½ cup	14.2	147	1
w/vinaigrette	½ cup	3.0	78	1
gelatin salad w/fruit & cheese	½ cup	4.6	74	0
macaroni salad w/mayo	½ cup	12.8	200	1

Item	Serving	Total Fat (g)	Calories	Fiber (g)
pasta primavera salad	1 cup	5.9	149	3
potato salad				
German style	½ cup	3.5	140	1
w/mayo dressing	½ cup	11.5	189	1
salad bar items				
alfalfa sprouts	2 T	0	2	0
bacon bits	1 T	1.0	21	0
beets, pickled	2 T	0	18	0
broccoli, raw	2 T	0	3	0
carrots, raw	2 T	0	6	0
cheese, shredded	2 T	4.6	56	0
chickpeas	2 T	0.3	36	1
cottage cheese	½ cup	5.1	116	0
croutons	½ oz.	2.6	62	0
cucumber	2 T	0	2	0
eggs, cooked, chopped	2 T	1.9	27	0
lettuce	½ cup	0	4	0
mushrooms, raw	2 T	0	2	0
onion, raw	2 T	0.1	7	0
pepper, green, raw	2 T	0	3	0
potato salad	½ cup	10.3	179	0
tomato, raw	2 slices	0	2	0
seven-layer salad	1 cup	17.8	226	2
tabbouli salad	½ cup	9.5	173	3
taco salad w/taco sauce	1 cup	14.0	202	2
three-bean salad	½ cup	8.2	145	3
three-bean salad w/o oil	½ cup	0.2	90	3
Waldorf salad w/mayo	½ cup	12.7	157	2

Eating Diary

It's important to keep track of fat grams, calories, and fiber for 21 days if you want to make sure that you are following the program as closely as possible, especially if you are attempting to lose weight quickly with the Weight-Loss Express. A sample daily record is reproduced here. You can photocopy this form as many times as you like, or simply keep track of the information required in a small notebook that fits in your pocket.

If you are following the Weight-Loss Express, the upper limit for daily fat grams is 30 for women and 40 for men; the calorie limits are 1200 for women and 1800 for men.[2] If you are simply trying to maintain your

[2]On a 1200-calorie diet, 27 grams of fat would equal 20 percent of calories, but for convenience I have rounded up to 30, assuming that 1200 calories amounts to a temporary restriction for most people, and that caloric requirements as well as fat intake will be higher on a maintenance diet.

weight, estimate your caloric needs from the table on the next page and set your fat-gram goal at 20 percent of total calories. The minimum daily goal for fiber is 25 grams, and 35 is better once your system becomes used to more roughage.

DAILY EATING DIARY

Date_____ Daily goals: Fat grams_____ Calories_____ Fiber_____

Food	Amount	Fat Grams	Calories	Fiber
Breakfast				
Lunch				
Dinner				
Snacks				
Total for today:				

GRAMS OF FAT THAT EQUAL 20 PERCENT
OF TOTAL CALORIES

Total Calories	Grams of Fat
1200	27
1300	29
1400	31
1500	33
1600	36
1700	38
1800	40
1900	42
2000	44
2100	47
2200	49
2300	51
2400	53
2500	56
2600	58
2700	60

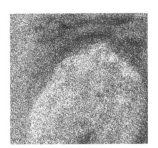

Index

Page numbers in **boldface** refer to recipes.
Page numbers in *italics* refer to tables.

definition of, 8
free radicals and, 10
in the home, 209–11
mechanism of, 9
protective phytochemicals vs., 22
vitamins and, 38–39
in workplace, 212
carcinomas, 5
cardiovascular disease, xiii, xiv
and altered form of LDL, 15
aspirin and, 199
cancer's similarities to, 11, 16–17
cholesterol as risk factor for, 13, 14
foam cells and, 15
herbs as preventives of, 193–95
lifestyle and, 12
mortality rates for, 12, 18
protective foods and, 52
saturated fat and, 12–13, 14, 16
smoking and, 12, 209
weight and, xvii
women and, 72
carotenoids, 27, 30
as antioxidants, 16
cancer-suppressing properties of, 24
carrot(s):
cabbage, green pepper and raisin salad,
106–7
and celery, 168
rainbow salad, 110–11
rosemary, 167
and shredded cabbage salad, 109
casserole(s):
barley/pine-nut, 141–42
green bean, 172
potato-tofu, 154
seafood, stove-top, 124
southwest, 131
soybean and lima, 144–45
spinach, 170–71
tuna, 130
cataracts, weight and, xvii, 72
catechins (tannins), 27, 30
cauliflower:
Burneta's millet mash, 143
curried squash/soup, 97–98
du Barry, 163–64
dusty, 164
celery:
and carrots, 168
soup, 96
Center for Science in the Public Interest,
184–85, 194

Centers for Disease Control, U.S., 189
chamomile, 197
chaparral, 197
cheese:
dark chocolate cheesecake, 180
Dave's rich and zesty burritos, 137–38
Dave's rich and zesty tostados, 138–39
escarole torte, 130–31
green-bean casserole, 172
green-bean ragout, 171
mock lasagna, 145–46
onion quiche, 132
Parmesan-dill Brussels sprouts, 165–66
southwest casserole, 131
spaghetti with tomatoes, basil and capers,
147–48
spinach casserole, 170–71
spinach lasagna, 148–49
stuffed winter squash, 133
cheesecake, dark chocolate, 180
chemoprotective phytochemicals, 30–34
chewy cocoa cake, 179
chicken:
broiled, with yogurt, 125–26
chard and rice soup, 100
curried spinach and, 126–27
Monna's white chili, 134–35
oven-fried, 129
oven-stewed, and vegetables, 127–28
rice and artichoke salad, 115–16
salad, tarragon, with vermicelli, 113
southwest casserole, 131
chickpea(s):
couscous and vegetables, 139–40
and potatoes, curried, 162–63
tuna with, 117
chili, Monna's white, 134–35
chili tomatoes and black beans, 143–44
chilled tomato-orange soup with avocado, 99
chocolate:
brownies, 177
chewy cocoa cake, 179
dark, cheesecake, 180
frosting, quick, 179–80
cholesterol, serum:
HDL, 14, 15
influences on level of, 13, 14
LDL, 13–16
level of daily, 46
as risk factor for cardiovascular disease, 16
chowder, clam, 96–97
chromium picolinate, 197
clam chowder, 96–97

coenzyme Q10, *197*
coffee cake, whole wheat, **176**
cold cucumber soup, **98**
comfrey, *197*
Commission E, 194*n*
confetti pasta with fish and artichokes, **148**
corn:
   -cakes, **94**
   Mexican quinoa salad, **116**
   rainbow salad, **110**
   stuffed winter squash, **133**
   tamale pie, **133–34**
counters, fat, 45, 78
couscous:
   chickpeas and vegetables, **139–40**
   salad, Greek, **114–15**
crab-meat and artichoke salad, **118**
creamy cabbage, **166**
creamy tofu dressing, **105**
Creole stew, **158**
cucumber:
   cabbage/tomato salad, **110**
   soup, cold, **98**
curried:
   chicken and spinach, **126–27**
   chickpeas and potatoes, **162–63**
   squash/cauliflower soup, **97–98**
   tofu and cabbage, **154–55**

dairy products, 48
dark chocolate cheesecake, **180**
Dave's hearty meat sauce, **174**
Dave's rich and zesty burritos, **137–38**
Dave's rich and zesty tostados, **138–39**
deep muscular relaxation, stress and, 208
desserts, 61, 62, **174–81**
diary, eating, 63–*64*, 78
diet(s), ix
   cancer risks and, 21, 22, 26
   cardiovascular disease and, 12–13
   cholesterol level and, 14
   disease prevention and, 3–4, 11, 16, 26
   failure of quick-weight-loss, xviii, xix
   quiz, 43
   typical American, xiv–xv, 18, 21–22, 44, 46,
     47, 200
Diet, The T-Factor (Katahn), 45, 79
dill-Parmesan Brussels sprouts, **165–66**
dinner, 59–63
   generic, 61–63
   steps to implementing cancer prevention
     good health diet at, 59–61
disease prevention:

aspirin and, 199
   diet and, 3–4, 11, 16
   herbs and, 193–96, 199
   lifestyle and, 3
   U.S.D.A. food pyramid and, 55
disease resistance, moderate physical activity
   and, 202
dithiothiones, cancer-blocking qualities of, 23
DNA (deoxyribonucleic acid), 7, 8, 15, 23, 24
   plant, 25
du Barry, cauliflower, **163–64**
dusty cauliflower, **164**

echinacea, *197*
   as immunostimulant, 195
   and treatment of infections, 196
eggplant salad, **112**
electromagnetic fields, 209, 211
electrophilic molecules, 9, 11, 22, 23
   see also free radicals
eleuthero ("Siberian ginseng"), 195
Enid's quick fruit pie, **178**
environmental pollutants:
   cancer and, 6, 7, 8
   free radicals and, 10
   in the home, 209–11
   and oxidative stress, 11
   vitamin C as antidote to, 38
   in workplace, 212
Environmental Protection Agency (EPA), 209,
   210
   Safe Drinking Water Hotline of, 211
enzymes, phytochemicals and, 22, 26
Ephedra (ma huang), *197*
escarole torte, **130–31**
ethnic food, cancer prevention good health diet
   and, 66–70

fat:
   consumption level of, 46, 55, 79
   counters, 45, 78
   dietary limitations on, 47–48
   and "no-fat" foods, 81–82
   quick weight loss and, 77–79
feverfew, *197*
fiber, 23, 24
   elimination rate of, 81
   lunchtime consumption of, 57–58
   recommended daily consumption of, 46,
     47
fish, 48, 50, 60, 61, **120–24**
   baked swordfish, **122**
   confetti pasta with artichokes and, **148**

Raisins (*continued*)
    cabbage, carrot and green pepper salad, **106–7**
    caramel brownies, **175**
    rainbow salad, **110**
Recommended Daily Allowance (RDA), 186, 188, 189, 200
red meat, 18
    in cancer prevention good health diet, 48
    cancer risks and, 20–21
    cutting consumption of, 50
    and Harvard School of Public Health study, 20
restaurants, 58, 66
rice:
    brown, with garlic, **139**
    chicken, and artichoke salad, **115–16**
    chicken, chard and, soup, **100**
    southwest casserole, **131**
roast(ed):
    onion salad, **107**
    pork tenderloin, **119–20**
    poultry, Tandoori style, **128–29**
    rosemary potatoes, **162**
    vegetables, **169**
rosemary:
    carrots, **167**
    potatoes, roasted, **162**

salad, **105–118**
    artichoke and crab-meat, **118**
    broccoli, **106**
    cabbage, carrot, green pepper and raisin, **106–7**
    chicken, rice and artichoke, **115–16**
    cucumber/cabbage/tomato, **110**
    eggplant, **112**
    Greek couscous, **114–15**
    main-course Greek, **108**
    Mexican quinoa, **116–17**
    pasta, **114**
    pickled beets, **111**
    rainbow, **110–11**
    roasted onion, **107**
    shredded cabbage and carrot, **109**
    tarragon chicken, with vermicelli, **113**
    three-bean, **109**
    tuna with chickpeas, **117**
salad dressing, **103–5**
    basic vinaigrette, **103–4**
    creamy tofu, **105**
    garlic vinaigrette, **104**
    lemon and garlic, **104–5**

salmon, teriyaki, **122–23**
salt, herb, **183**
sarcomas, 5
saturated fat:
    and cancer, 9, 18–19
    and cardiovascular disease, 13, 14, 16
sauce, Dave's hearty meat, **174**
sauté, tri-color pepper, **169–70**
savory turkey loaf, **135–36**
saw palmetto, *198–99*
scalloped potatoes and tofu, **153**
scurvy, 35
seafood:
    artichoke and crab-meat salad, **118**
    clam chowder, **96–97**
    stove-top casserole, **124**
    see also fish
seasonings, **181–83**
selenium, 24, 40
servings, U.S.D.A. food pyramid and, *53, 54*
setpoint, xviii–xix
shark cartilage, *199*
shredded cabbage and carrot salad, **109**
simple masala, **181–82**
simple pot of beans, **137**
Smith, Manuel J., 205
smoking:
    cancer and, 8–9, 209
    cardiovascular disease and, 12, 209
snacks, 51, 52, 62
soft drinks, 48
soup, **95–102**
    beet and cabbage borscht, **101**
    celery, **96**
    chicken, chard and rice, **100**
    chilled tomato-orange with avocado, **99**
    clam chowder, **96–97**
    cold cucumber, **98**
    curried squash/cauliflower, **97–98**
    of the day, **95–96**
    gazpacho primo, **102**
    mushroom, **100–101**
southwest casserole, **131**
soybean and lima casserole, **144–45**
spaghetti with tomatoes, basil and capers, **147**
spiced tofu loaf, **156**
spices and herbs, 89–91
spinach:
    casserole, **170–71**
    curried chicken and, **126–27**
    lasagna, **148–49**
    Mediterranean-style, **170**
    orange roughy with, **123**